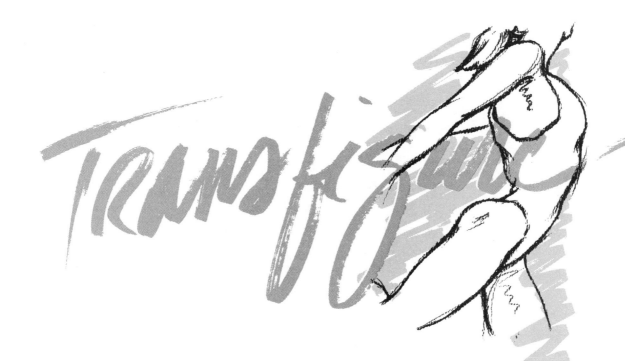

Transfigure

VOLUME II

FOR THE

ULTIMATE

UPPER BODY

• Health For Life •

Also from
Health For Life:

Transfigure:
For the Ultimate Buttocks & Thighs

Legendary Abs II

Power ForeArms!

Maximum Calves

The Human Fuel Handbook
Nutrition for Peak Athletic Performance

SynerAbs II: 6 Minutes to a Flatter Stomach

SynerShape: A Scientific Weight Loss Guide

SynerStretch: For Total Body Flexibility

The Psychology of Weight Loss:
A Guided Introspection

Secrets of Advanced Bodybuilders
*A manual of synergistic weight training
for the whole body*

ISBN 0-944831-24-9
Library of Congress Catalog Card #90-83827

Health For Life
8033 Sunset Blvd., Suite 483, Los Angeles, CA 90046, (213) 306-0777

CREDITS AND ACKNOWLEDGEMENTS

Book design and illustration by Irene DiConti McKinniss;
photography by Michael Neveux; photo styling by
Sharon Crabtree; model: Teal Roberts.

Special thanks to Andrew Shields M.D., Marylou Taylor,
M.S., and Chris Paredes for their expertise and their
suggestions throughout the development of the
Transfigure II program.

Additional thanks to Stevan Walton, D.C.

contents

WHAT
TRANSFIGURE II
WILL DO
FOR YOU

Transfigure II *is a scientifically designed formula for producing a toned, shapely upper body. Based on extensive biomechanical research and analysis, this course targets the major muscle groups that determine the shape of the arms, shoulders and chest.*

Transfigure II *uses fast, intense triceps routines to firm and tone the upper arms, and extensive pectoral routines to fill in the upper chest and create support for the breasts. Exercises for the biceps, shoulders, and back are also included to ensure symmetry and balanced development.*

*Like its companion course **Transfigure: For Ultimate Thighs and Buttocks**, **Transfigure II** delivers maximum results in minimum time, without employing potentially injurious exercise techniques.*

The fact is, efficient training is a rarity. *The muscle conditioning exercises in aerobic classes are seldom adjusted for optimum form, rep numbers, pace, sequence—details that have a major impact on the effectiveness of a program. Routines published in most magazines tend simply to perpetuate common misunderstandings.*

Transfigure II *takes a fresh look at what women want, æsthetically, and at the scientific basis for achieving it. Using proven biomechanical principles, this program selects the most effective exercises and combines them into an efficient, balanced program.*

*This high-gear system of upper body work is guaranteed to give you the sleek, bodyshaped contour you want. Whether you're aiming at general firmness and tone, or strength and high definition, you'll find in **Transfigure II** a concise, powerful means to achieve your goal!*

TRAINING THEORY:
What and Why

CHAPTER ONE

A Word
About
Fat Loss

Surveys show many women are not content with the appearance of their upper arms. The much-lamented loose, flabby upper arm is generally caused by two factors, both of which you can control.

First is a lack of tone in the muscles of the upper arm—especially the <u>triceps</u>, which defines the back of the arm. **Transfigure II** *is a dynamic means of conditioning these contour-determining muscles, among others.*

In many cases, however, there is also excess <u>fat</u> in the picture. *Even small amounts of fat can obscure what muscle definition you do have.*

Fat is nothing more than stored energy. To reduce excess fat anywhere on your body, you must create a <u>calorie deficit</u> to use up that energy. This is done by performing <u>aerobic exercise</u> while <u>moderately restricting your caloric intake</u>. Net result: you burn more energy than you consume, and fat stores shrink.*

Despite the popularity of "spot reducing" approaches, only sustained effort involving many major muscle groups will burn enough calories to significantly mobilize fat stores.

Most effective in this regard is continuous exercise performed three to five times a week, <u>burning at least 300</u>

---

* For complete guidelines on fat metabolism, see *SynerShape: A Scientific Weight Loss Guide*, available from *Health For Life*.

calories per session. *Moderate-intensity exercise (where your pulse rate stays at 60 to 70% of your maximum) should be sustained for 30 to 45 minutes. Walking, cycling, lap swimming, and low-impact dancing are good moderate-intensity activities that place minimal stress on the joints. More strenuous forms of aerobic activity—running, stair climbing, rope jumping, cross-country skiing—are acceptable if you can do them continuously for at least 20 minutes.*

Does it matter whether you do moderate or high-intensity exercise? Current research suggests it doesn't.* *In the end,* **whether from 20 minutes of strenuous exercise or 40 minutes of moderate exercise, the number of calories burned is the only concern.**

Criteria for the ideal fat-burning routine:

▲ *Low-to-moderate-intensity exercise (60 to 70% of your maximum) for 30 to 45 minutes,* <u>or</u>

▲ *High-intensity exercise (80% of maximum) for 20 minutes*

▲ *3 to 5 workouts per week*

▲ *Low-impact movements to minimize joint stress*

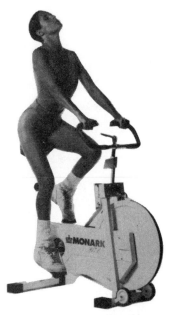

Fig. 1—If you want to lose fat, there's no way around needing to burn more calories than you take in. The balance of *calories consumed in food against calories expended in activity* is what determines fat loss.

---

* During low-intensity, long-duration exercise, the body draws most of its calories from fat, whereas during brief, high-intensity exercise it draws most of its calories from glycogen, a storage form of sugar. Although it might sound as if you could preferentially remove calories from fat stores by doing longer stretches of low-intensity exercise, in fact, you can't, because the depleted stores get replenished.

CHAPTER TWO

Aerobics Classes: Aerobic vs. Muscular Conditioning

Aerobic dance classes
have become the activity
of choice for women
wishing to lose weight and
develop cardiovascular
fitness and muscle tone.
This chapter discusses the
pros and cons of aerobic
dance in relation to these
goals.

Aerobic dance* has made regular exercise attractive to
many people who otherwise wouldn't exercise at all.
However, the standard aerobics class format attempts to
blend together <u>aerobic</u> conditioning (important for
cardiovascular fitness and fat reduction) with <u>muscle</u>
conditioning (for shape and definition)—an attempt that

---

* meaning *aerobic dance classes or routines*, which combine forms of
aerobic exercise with muscle-conditioning exercises.

unfortunately limits its ability to achieve either one with optimum efficiency. These are two very different types of conditioning ideally involving separate training modalities.

As a rule, the "aerobic" portion of most classes—the cardiovascular training—delivers pretty good value. The "toning" portion, on the other hand, generally does not, for two reasons:

Poor Targeting. No amount of determination can make a muscle respond if it's not _involved_ in the movement being performed. Strange as this may sound, it applies to a number of commonly-performed exercises. Poor targeting can be corrected by evaluating the exercise in question in relation to the natural action of the muscle it aims to work. (See page 13.)

Low-Resistance, High-Repetitions. Many popular upper-body toning exercises involve such extremely low resistance that they necessitate astronomical numbers of repetitions. It's not unusual to see students performing 50 or more reps of certain movements.

This widespread mania for high-rep, low-resistance conditioning exercise stems from a pair of widely held misconceptions: First, that using more resistance will render you overly muscular (not true), and second, that high-rep, low-resistance arm exercises offer significant aerobic benefit (also not true). These misconceptions are so ingrained that many students _expect_ to do high reps, and may even feel shortchanged if they don't. Nevertheless, the facts are:

> ▼ **Low-rep, _high_-resistance is the fastest way to achieve muscle tone _or_ growth, and it affords complete control over how muscular you become.**

> ▼ **In most cases, toning exercises do not involve enough muscle groups or enough resistance to tax the cardiovascular system**

significantly; i.e., <u>they are not</u>
<u>efficient for aerobic</u>
<u>conditioning or losing weight</u>.

*While genuine aerobic exercise is useful and necessary for cardiovascular fitness and weight control, **the most** **efficient way to tone muscle is with a <u>separate</u> <u>high-resistance routine</u>** specifically aimed at muscle conditioning.*

HOW *TRANSFIGURE* FIGURES IN

Transfigure II *employs efficiently targeted, high-resistance exercises to deliver muscle development you won't get in a standard aerobic workout.*

*We strongly recommend performing regular aerobic exercise—of whatever type you choose—for the cardiovascular training and calorie burning it provides. If you are involved in an aerobics class, the minimal amount of upper-body toning work included there can serve as a warm up for performing the **Transfigure II** routine.*

Note: *If you are involved in a **muscle-conditioning** class in which substantial time (15-30 minutes per session) is devoted to upper-body toning exercises, then you do, if you wish, have the option of using the information in this book simply to fine-tune your existing routine. This will improve your results and help you avoid the potentially injurious motions in many standard exercises.*

*For optimum results, however, we recommend the **Transfigure II** routines <u>in place of</u> any other upper-body toning exercises. By all means, continue to perform aerobic work aimed at fat reduction and cardiovascular conditioning—but follow it with the appropriate **Transfigure II** routine for upper-body muscle conditioning. This will guarantee the greatest possible return on your investment of time and effort.*

TRAINING ALERT

THE "M" WORD

Many women, when undertaking physical conditioning, are concerned that they not develop an obviously <u>muscular</u> look. They categorically avoid all exercises involving weights or muscular overloading for fear of mutating suddenly into some sort of Amazonian can-crusher.

*The fact is, whether you're aiming for a firm, slender shape or a bodybuilder's physique, it's still a matter of **conditioning muscle**—the difference is simply one of degree. The purpose of this course is to help you achieve any degree of muscular development, definition, and growth you choose.*

A radical increase in size, <u>if</u> that were your goal, would occur over a long period of time, involving progressive resistance and a lot of hard work. If you want a bodybuilder's physique, this program includes separate high-intensity routines to help you achieve that goal. Otherwise, rest assured that extreme muscularity never occurs "accidentally!"

Fig. 2—Toned and slender or bodybuilder-chiseled, you have complete control over how developed your muscles become.

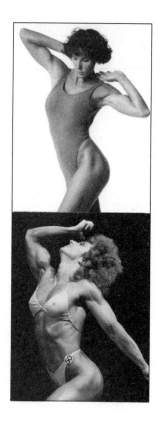

CHAPTER THREE

Muscle:
the Raw
Material

Muscle serves a number of
purposes, both in
protecting and animating
the body. It is also the
essential æsthetic element
adorning the human frame.
Muscle tissue is the lean
clay from which the human
form is molded.

Several muscle groups are of particular concern in
creating an aesthetically pleasing upper body. A firm,
"filled in" upper chest, for instance, is the result of pectoral
development—particularly that of the upper pectorals.
The lines of the upper arm are enhanced by a pair of
muscles: the triceps in back, and the biceps in front.
Finally, the shoulders are shaped by the deltoid muscles.

Training these muscle groups with the goal of creating
firm, shapely upper-body contour is the primary aim of the
routines to follow.

Balanced Development. At each joint, muscle groups
work against one another in pairs to provide stability.
Since most daily movements involve these pairs working

together, it is best from a health standpoint to train both groups of each pair.

For instance, the biceps and triceps act, respectively, to bend and straighten the elbow. Even if you are more concerned with toning the backs of the arms, it's important to do at least some biceps work for the sake of elbow joint stability.

Likewise, the chest and upper back act, respectively, to pull the arms forward and back. Even if you are more concerned with toning your chest, it's important to do some work for the upper back muscles.

In addition to the health benefits, working for balanced development will help you achieve a symmetrical, beautifully contoured appearance.

FORM AND FUNCTION

Each of the muscles covered in this course acts on the shoulder or elbow in a characteristic way. Familiarity with the specific actions of these muscles enables you to assess the effectiveness of any exercise. In simplest terms, **to be effective, an exercise must mimic the action of its intended target muscle.**

Slight changes of body position can drastically shift focus away from the target muscle. This shift renders a movement essentially useless. Unforunately, it also makes it easier, allowing you to do more repetitions—and that's psychologically reinforcing, habituating the body to the ineffective motion.

The Sixth Sense. One of the most useful things for any active person to develop is a kinæsthetic sense of the muscle groups and their functions. This means being able to associate the position and motion of your limbs with physical sensations in the muscles, tendons, and joints. (Did you ever wonder, for instance, how you're able to scratch your nose in the dark? This is accomplished using *kinæsthetic awareness.) Combine this awareness with a basic understanding of anatomy, and you have an invaluable, <u>built-in</u> training resource!*

The following table illustrates basic anatomical information that will help you tune in, kinæsthetically, to the movements of the exercises to come.

Pectoralis Major (Chest) — *A fan-shaped muscle spreading inward from the upper arm to the collar and breast bones. When contracted, it pulls the arm across the chest at one of several angles, depending on which segment of the muscle is active.*

▲ **Upper Pectoral**—*pulls the arm <u>up</u> across the chest*

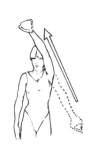
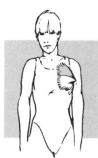

Pulls arm up across the chest

Upper Pectoral

▲ **Middle Pectoral**—*pulls the arms <u>straight</u> across the chest*

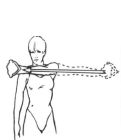
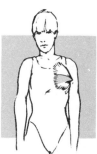

Pulls arm straight across the chest

Middle Pectoral

▲ **Lower Pectoral**—*pulls the arms <u>down</u> across the chest*

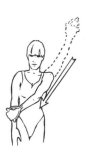
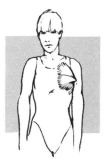

Pulls arm down across the chest

Lower Pectoral

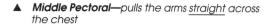

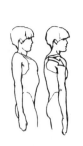
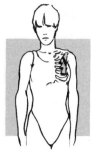

Pulls shoulder blade down and forward

Pectoralis Minor

Pectoralis Minor — *Lies underneath the pectoralis major. Pulls the shoulder blade <u>down and forward</u>.*

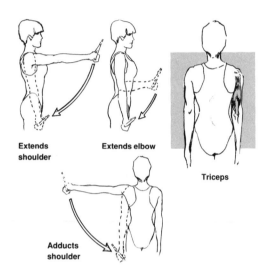

Extends shoulder

Extends elbow

Adducts shoulder

Triceps

Triceps — *Straight, 3-headed muscle that <u>extends, or straightens, the elbow</u>. One head, the long head, also <u>extends and adducts the shoulder</u> (it brings the arm down from the front, and pulls it toward the body from the side).*

Upper Back

▲ *Latissmus Dorsi*—Fan-shaped muscle running from the front of the upper arm, underneath the shoulder, spreading out as it wraps around the side of the torso to attach to the spine. <u>Pulls the arm down and toward the rear.</u>

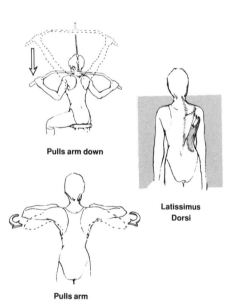

Pulls arm down

Latissimus Dorsi

Pulls arm toward rear

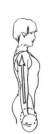

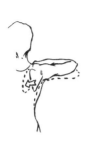

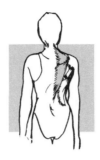

**Raises or lowers
shoulders**

**Pulls scapulae in
toward spine**

Trapezius

▲ **Trapezius**—*Trapezoid-shaped muscle whose
fibers spread from the shoulder to the center line,
attaching along the spine from the middle back
to the base of the skull. Depending on which
portion contracts, can* <u>*raise or lower the
shoulders*</u>*, or* <u>*draw the shoulder blades in toward
the spine*</u>*.*

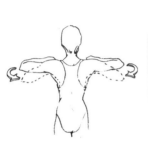

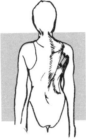

**Pull upper arm
toward scapula**

**Teres Major
Teres Minor,
Infraspinatus**

▲ **Teres Major, Teres Minor, Infraspinatus**—*3 small,
straight muscles running from the upper arm to
the scapula (shoulder blade). Among other
functions, they* <u>*pull the upper arm toward the
scapula*</u>*.*

Lower Back

▲ **Spinal Erectors**—*A group of muscles that run
vertically along the spine. They* <u>*extend, or
straighten, the back*</u>*.*

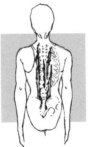

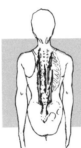

Straighten back

Spinal Erectors

Biceps — *a straight, 2-headed muscle running along the front of the upper arm.*

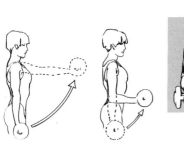

Flexes shoulder

Bends elbow

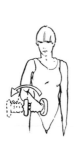

Biceps, Long Head

▲ **Long Head**—*bends the elbow and raises the arm forward at the shoulder*

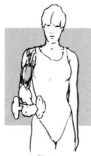

Supinates arm

Biceps, Short Head

▲ **Short Head**—*also supinates the forearm (rotates it outward)*

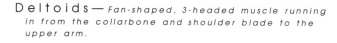

Deltoids—*Fan-shaped, 3-headed muscle running in from the collarbone and shoulder blade to the upper arm.*

▲ **Anterior (Front) Deltoid**—*raises the arm to the front and rotates it inward*

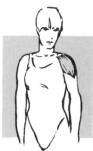
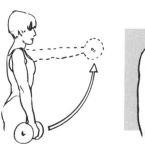

Raises arm to the front   Front Delt

▲ **Lateral (Side) Deltoid**—*raises the arm to the side*

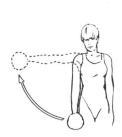
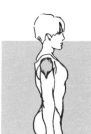
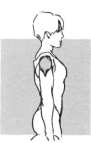

Raises arm to the side   Side Delt

▲ **Posterior (Rear) Deltoid**—*raises the arm toward the rear and rotates it outward*

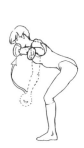
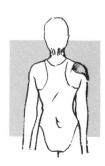

Raises arm to the rear
Rotates arm outward   Rear Delt

Four Steps to Efficient Training

This chapter explains four basic points of effective training. It's not necessary to develop a detailed understanding of biomechanical principles to use *Transfigure II*. On the other hand, knowing some of the basic theory behind efficient training will help sharpen your mental focus and improve your results.

STEP ONE: DEFINE YOUR GOALS

Most specific conditioning goals fall into one of two general categories: performance or appearance. **Your goal dictates your training strategy.** *Training methods appropriate for various goals may overlap in some respects but differ in others. That's why no program can be maximally efficient until you've decided exactly what you're working for.*

The **Transfigure II** program is designed to enhance appearance: specifically, _to improve muscle tone and contour_.

Tone is the degree to which your muscles remain contracted when you relax. Good muscle tone gives the body a youthful, fit appearance. Muscle **contour** is a function of muscle size.

Our training strategy, therefore, places less emphasis on building extreme strength and explosive power, and more emphasis on improving muscle contour through increases in muscle size. Most women require only small size increases to shape underdeveloped muscles.*

Since the recommendations for size training and strength training overlap in many respects, training aimed at muscle appearance _will_ produce an increase in strength and athletic facility. However, it is not the intention of this course to create a training program aimed _primarily_ at substantial strength/performance gains.

STEP TWO: TARGETING

Targeting means matching the motion of an exercise to the action of a specific muscle. **The more precisely you target a muscle, the less time and effort it takes to train it.**

Good targeting requires first understanding what a given muscle does, and then, through exact body positioning and alignment, using it to do _precisely that_, with as little assistance as possible from other muscles.

. . . .

* The exception would be the bodybuilder, for whom substantial development is essential for symmetry. To achieve this requires a program of graduated resistance like that described in the upper levels of the Expanded routines in the Program section.

For instance, Butterflies (Fig. 3), a common exercise that supposedly targets the triceps, involves a very short-arc flutter of the arms at the sides.

In fact, the triceps (whose primary function is to straighten the elbow), are not involved at all in this movement. What little work is being done here is being done by muscles of the back (working against practically no resistance—see next section). The isometric contraction of the triceps keeping the arms straight is of minimal value.

Exercises like the Butterfly are badly conceived and best eliminated from your routine. There are many instances, however, of well-designed exercises that depend on minute adjustments of form to make them effectively work their target muscles. Many of these important adjustments are featured in the "wrong" illustrations in the Exercise section to follow.

The corrections in body position mentioned throughout this course, tiny as they may seem, can have a huge impact on efficiency. It pays to be meticulous about exercise form.

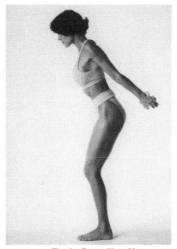

Fig. 3—Butterflies: Movement involves muscles of the upper back, not the triceps

STEP THREE: HIGH RESISTANCE

There is no reason to do hundreds of reps! In fact, there's reason not to:

Although simple muscle <u>toning</u> will occur as a result of almost any muscular activity, <u>shaping</u>—creating new contours—requires subtle increases in muscle size, which the muscle must be overloaded to achieve. This overload can <u>only</u> occur with low-rep, high-resistance training.

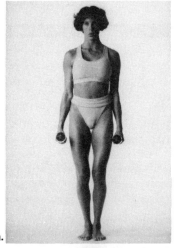

a.

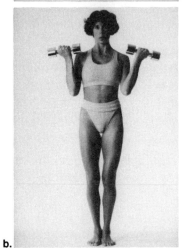

b.

▼ *Tone develops from muscle activity of any kind—but it develops <u>faster</u> from high-resistance work*

▼ *Shape (size increase) develops from muscular overload; this can <u>only</u> be accomplished using high resistance*

Any motion using weights or machines is potentially a high-resistance exercise. Bodyweight movements, on the other hand, may or may not provide adequate resistance, depending on the body's position.

Pom-Poms, (Fig. 4), for example, present some interesting problems. Performed without weights, as they often are, they are inefficient because the arms simply don't weigh enough to overload the muscles. On the other hand, performed with dumbbells, they have the potential to strain the shoulder and elbow joints because of the rotation involved. This is a no-win exercise.

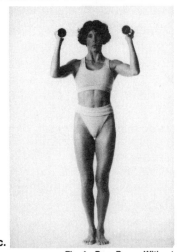

c.

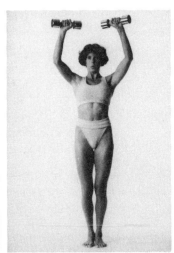

d.

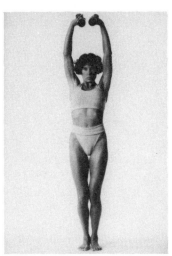

e.

Fig. 4—Pom-Poms: Without weights, they offer insufficient resistance; with weights, they can stress joints

Doing hundreds of reps of a less-efficient exercise may eventually build muscle tone, but you can tone *and* shape in a fraction of the time simply by increasing resistance. **Transfigure II** 's exercises are designed so that, on average, 8 to 10 repetitions will be sufficient to create an overload.

STEP FOUR: LOW INJURY POTENTIAL

Some upper-body exercises have the potential to place damaging stress on the elbows, shoulders, and lower back. A prime consideration in the creation of this course has been to minimize those stresses.

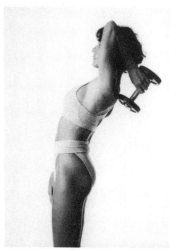

In some cases, joint stress can be reduced by a simple adjustment of form. Standing Triceps Extensions (Fig. 5), for instance, are often performed with an arched back. Arching the back adds nothing to the effectiveness of the exercise and can, in time, lead to chronic lower-back pain. Standing Triceps Extensions are just as effective, and far safer, without the arch.

Throughout this course, whenever possible, we will describe similar adjustments to minimize possible joint strain.

Fig. 5—Standing Triceps Extensions: Arched back stresses lower vertebrae

REVIEW—FOUR POINTS OF EFFECTIVE TRAINING

Step 1: Set specific goals

- ▲ *Goals determine training method*
- ▲ *Enhancing appearance requires toning and small size increases to create contour and definition.*

Step 2: Targeting

- ▲ *Effective exercises mimic the action of their target muscles, while requiring as little help as possible from other muscles.*

Step 3: Resistance

- ▲ *The fastest and most effective way to tone and shape is by using high resistance and few reps.*

Step 4: Low injury potential

- ▲ *Upper -body exercises have the potential to strain the lower back, elbows, and shoulders.*
- ▲ *Transfigure II will demonstrate how to reduce the danger in many cases by making minor modifications to exercise form.*

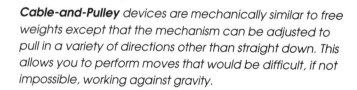

T R A I N I N G
A L E R T

R E S I S T A N C E   D E V I C E S

The routines in this course offer you certain exercise options, based on the equipment available to you. We offer here a description of different types of resistance devices, along with a discussion of their relative merits.

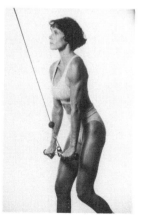

Fig. 6—Push-Up Handles

Bodyweight means just that: pushing or pulling your body against the force of gravity. Many of the bodyweight exercises in this course, because of their particular leverage characteristics, are excellent high-resistance exercises.

Push-Up Handles, though not themselves a "resistance device," can be used to increase the range of motion of standard triceps and chest exercises, increasing their effectiveness. They also eliminate the potentially damaging wrist stress associated with standard Push-Ups.

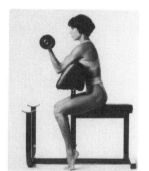

Fig. 7—Free Weights: barbells
and dumbbells

Free Weights are standard barbells and dumbbells. The weights are held in the hands. Free-weights always pull straight down, in the direction of gravity. Free weight exercises involve placing the body in a variety of positions, enabling different muscles to work directly against the resistance.

Cable-and-Pulley devices are mechanically similar to free weights except that the mechanism can be adjusted to pull in a variety of directions other than straight down. This allows you to perform moves that would be difficult, if not impossible, working against gravity.

Both free weights and cable-and-pulley devices allow you considerable freedom of movement. The advantage of

Fig. 8—Cable-and-Pulley

this freedom is that it allows you to make subtle adjustments in body position to obtain optimum targeting with minimum joint strain.

*Another advantage is that, in many cases, these devices make demands on muscles other than the target muscle to <u>stabilize</u> the body—that is, to hold it in position while you perform the exercise. This promotes **functional strength**, an integration of muscle group function that helps the body meet everyday strength demands. Functional strength is a very useful byproduct of physical conditioning.*

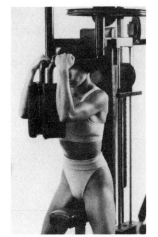

Fig. 9—Example of cam machine

Machines *(such as <u>Nautilus</u>, <u>Icarian</u>, <u>Universal</u>, <u>Eagle</u>, and others) take the job of holding the body in position away from the stabilizing muscles. Machines are therefore less effective at generating functional strength than their free-weight equivalents. On the other hand, machines can be extremely valuable for isolating individual muscles or muscle segments. They also enable you to use higher poundages safely when you don't have a partner to spot you (for example, when doing the Bench Press).*

Machines have one other advantage over free weights: they're harder to use incorrectly. If you're a beginner, the forced guidance they provide trains proper movement patterns into your nervous system and helps you get the feel of using specific muscles.

Despite the advantages and convenience of machines, however, it's best to include some free-weight exercises in your routine for the functional strength benefits they provide.

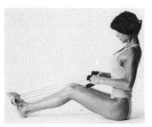

Fig. 10—Elastic Bands

Elastic bands*. The strap pictured in this course is called the <u>HFL Body Toner</u>, and is manufactured by Health For Life. It consists of a hollow rubber tube whose resistance and range of stretch are well suited for upper-body exercises. Three neoprene handles afford a secure grip and help reduce the risk of "slingshotting."*

Warning! To avoid injury when using any elastic bands:

▼ **Never place your head or face in line with a stretched elastic band**

▼ **Examine your bands frequently for signs of wear, especially where the elastic joins with any clasps or fasteners, and discontinue use at first signs of wear**

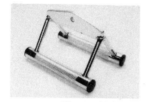

Fig . 11—V-Handle

V-Handle. Although not found in all gyms, the V-Handle is an extremely useful accessory for performing Close-Grip Pull-Ups, an advanced back exercise.

CHAPTER FIVE

How To
Use
The Transfigure II
Program

**The *Transfigure II* program
is divided into three
sections: *Exercises*,
Routines, and *Schedule*.**

EXERCISES

*This section contains all the exercises used in the
Transfigure II routines. Some exercises listed involve only
bodyweight; others incorporate light-resistance devices
such as dumbbells or elastic bands; most make use of
various machines found in gyms and sports clubs.*

ROUTINES

*There are two categories of routines to choose from:
<u>Condensed</u> and <u>Expanded</u>. The <u>Condensed</u> routines offer
an intense, quick way to shape your upper body. These
routines are ideal if you have limited time to train. The
<u>Expanded</u> routines are more flexible than the <u>Condensed</u>
ones and ultimately will produce greater improvement.
However, they take a bit more time to do.*

SCHEDULE

The routines are followed by general guidelines for scheduling your workouts using either the Condensed or Expanded approach.

THE
EXERCISES

This section describes how to perform all the exercises in the *Transfigure II* routines. The exercises are grouped according to the muscles they target.

In many cases, you will find two descriptions of an exercise, "Standard" and "Optimized." These call attention to the differences between the way an exercise is usually done and the *best* way to do it. Remember, the finepoints of form make a big difference.

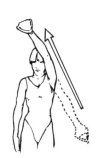

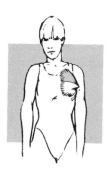

Pulls arm up across the chest

Upper Pec

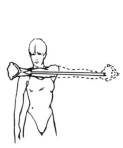

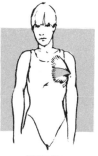

Pulls arm straight across the chest

Middle Pec

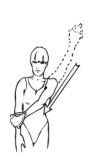

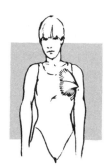

Pulls arm down across the chest

Lower Pec

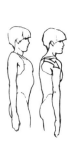

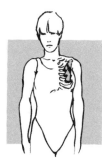

Pulls shoulder blade down and forward

Pec Minor

CHAPTER SIX

CHEST

The shape of the chest is determined by the **pectoralis major**, a fan-shaped muscle spreading inward from the upper arm to the collar and breast bones. When contracted, it <u>pulls the arm across the chest</u> at one of several angles, depending on which segment of the muscle is active.

▲ **Upper pectoral**—Pulls arm <u>up</u> across chest

▲ **Middle pectoral**—Pulls arm <u>straight</u> across chest

▲ **Lower pectoral**—Pulls arm <u>down</u> across chest

▲ Beneath the pectoralis major lies the **pectoralis minor**, whose function is to <u>pull the shoulder blade down and forward</u>, as when you hunch your shoulders. To involve both major and minor pectoral muscles, many of the exercises in this section will call for moving the arms forward (major) and hunching the shoulders (minor).

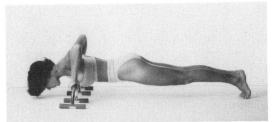

Fig. 12a—Elbows away from the body; targeting pecs

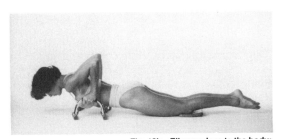

Fig. 12b—Elbows close to the body; targeting triceps

T R A I N I N G   A L E R T

P U S H - U P   T A R G E T I N G

Push-Ups is a very versatile exercise that can effectively made to target either the pectorals or the triceps. As with the Bench Press, the <u>narrower the hand position,</u> the greater the <u>triceps</u> contribution, the <u>wider the hand position</u>, the greater the <u>pectoral</u> contribution.

Since bodies vary, it's impossible to specify an ideal hand spread to focus on the pecs. But here are some guidelines:

▲ *Standard Push-Up width—hands just wider than shoulders—is effective for most people. Individuals with longer arms may need a wider spread.*

▲ *If you spread your arms far enough, eventually you'll feel the movement primarily in your delts.*

The key to targeting the <u>pecs</u> lies in moving the elbows <u>away from the body</u> as you descend (Fig. 12a). Conversely, keeping the elbows <u>close to the body</u> will target the <u>triceps</u> (Fig. 12b). The second form of Push-Up will be listed in the Triceps Chapter beginning page 47.

Push-Up Handles. *The effectiveness of most kinds of Push-Ups can be increased using Push-Up handles. These not only increase range of motion, allowing for more complete development, they also decrease your risk of developing <u>metacarpal tunnel syndrome</u>, a painful inflammation of the wrist. MTS can be brought on by the pressure that doing Push-Ups without Push-Up handles places on the wrists.*

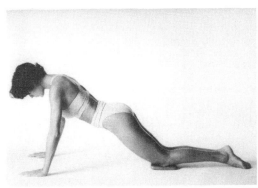

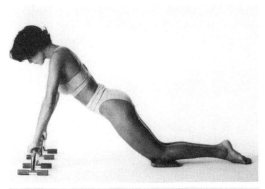

Fig. 13a, b—Elbows moving out to the side at about 45° angles

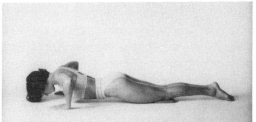

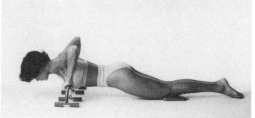

Fig. 13c, d—With handles; palms aimed back toward feet

KNEELING PUSH-UPS
target: pectorals

Standard Technique

Assume Kneeling Push-Up position, hands facing forward at about shoulder width. Bend at the elbows to lower your body. Reverse the motion and repeat.

Optimized Technique

Hand position during Kneeling Push-Ups is important not only for focusing on the target muscle, but also for minimizing potentially injurious stress on the wrists and elbows. Kneeling Push-Ups should always be done with the hands pointing straight forward or angled inward slightly. Angling them outward places unnecessary stress on your wrists.

Spread your hands slightly wider than your shoulders, and place them on the ground at the level of your upper chest (Fig. 13a). Keep your back rigid and your body straight as you slowly lower yourself until your chest touches the floor. Your elbows should move out to the sides at an angle of about 45 degrees (Fig. 13b).

Push yourself back up. At the top of the motion, make sure you roll the shoulders "forward" to fully engage the pectoralis minor. Repeat.

Using Push-Up Handles: *Follow the guidlines above. Position the handles so that your palms are aimed at your feet throughout the exercise (Fig. 13c,d). Don't allow your wrists to bend back or you defeat the purpose of using the handles.*

PUSH-UPS

target: pectorals, primarily middle pectorals

Standard Technique

Assume standard Push-Up position, hands facing forward at about shoulder width. Bend at the elbows to lower your body. Reverse the motion and repeat.

Optimized Technique

Hand position during Push-Ups is important not only for focusing on the target muscle, but also for minimizing potentially injurious stress on the wrists and elbows. Regular Push-Ups should always be done with the hands pointing straight forward or angled inward slightly. Angling them outward places unnecessary stress on your wrists.

Spread your hands slightly wider than your shoulders, and place them on the ground at the level of your upper chest (Fig. 14a).

Keep your back rigid and your body straight as you slowly lower yourself until your chest touches the floor. Your elbows should move out to the sides at an angle of about 45 degrees.

Push yourself back up (Fig. 14b). At the top of the motion, make sure you roll the shoulders "forward" to fully engage the pectoralis minor. Repeat.

Using Push-Up Handles: *Follow the guidlines above. Position the handles so that your palms are aimed at your feet throughout the exercise (Fig. 14c). Don't allow your wrists to bend back or you defeat the purpose of using the handles.*

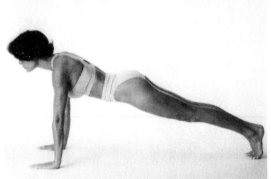

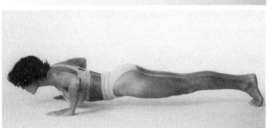

Fig. 14a, b—Elbows moving out to the side at about 45° angles

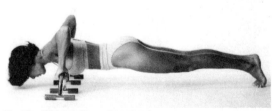

Fig. 14c—With handles; palms aimed back toward feet

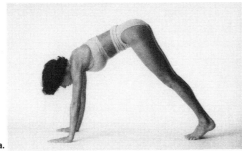

a.

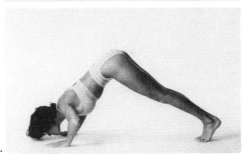

b.

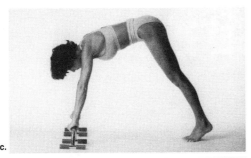

c.

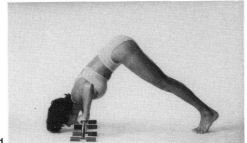

d.

TENT PUSH-UPS
target: pectorals, primarily upper pectorals

Placing your upper body on a <u>decline</u> during Push-Ups shifts shift the emphasis from mid to upper pecs.

Standard Technique

Beginning in standard Push-Up position, walk your feet forward, bending at the hips so your body assumes a jack-knife posture. Keep your knees and back straight. Bending at the elbows, lower your nose to the floor. Push up and repeat.

Optimized Technique

Perform as described above (Fig.15a,b). Your fingers should point straight forward or angle in slightly throughout the movement.

You can control the level of difficulty by varying how far forward you bring your feet—the farther forward, the higher the resistance experienced by the upper pecs.

Using Push-Up Handles: *Follow the guidelines above. The handles should be positioned slightly wider than shoulder width, with the bars in a straight line so that your palms face down to your feet (Fig. 15c,d).*

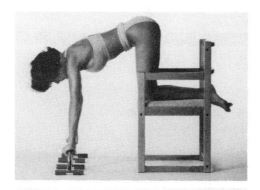

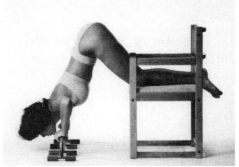

Fig. 16a, b—Optimum starting angle is between 45 and 60˚

DECLINE KNEELING PUSH-UPS
target: upper pectorals

Standard Technique

Kneel on the seat of a chair. Place your hands on the floor, shoulder width, at the level of your upper chest. Your fingers should point straight ahead or slightly to the sides. Lower your body until your nose touches the floor. Push up and repeat.

Optimized Technique

The steeper the angle of your upper body, the higher the resistance offered by the exercise—up to a point, at which the emphasis shifts off the pectorals and onto the front deltoids. The optimum angle for your body at the start of the exercise is between 45 and 60 degrees to the floor.

In the starting position, your arms should be vertical. This position will result in maximum stress through the upper pecs (Fig. 16a).

Lower your body until your nose touches the floor, keeping your back rigid (Fig. 16b). Push up and repeat.

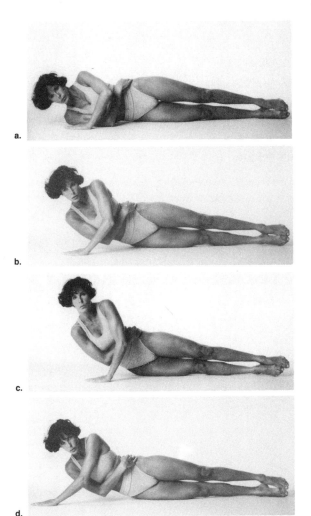

a.

b.

c.

d.

Fig. 17

ONE-ARM SIDE PUSH-UPS
target: upper pectorals

Lie on your left side on a soft pad, legs extended straight out. Rest your left hand on your right oblique (over the ribs at waist level). Place your right hand palm down on the floor in front of your face, fingers parallel to your body (Fig. 17a).

Concentrating on keeping your obliques relaxed, press your right hand against the floor to lift your torso. Your lower hip should remain on the pad. Feel for the tension in your upper right pectorals (Fig. 17b). Lower and repeat. Alternate sets on each side.

You can increase the resistance by planting your hand closer to your waist (Fig. 17c); you can decrease it by placing your hand closer to the top of your head (Fig. 17d).

Using Push-Up Handles: *Follow the guidelines above. The handle should be positioned at a 45-degree angle in front of your face.*

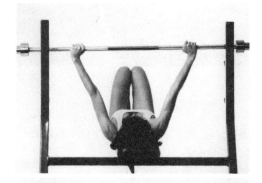

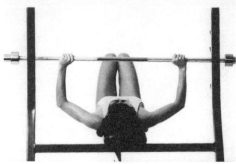

Fig. 18a, b—Grip width should be
wide enough that forearms don't
become parallel while
lowering the bar

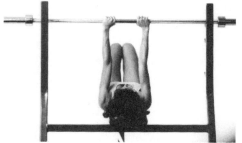

Fig. 18c—WRONG! Too narrow a grip

SUPINE BENCH PRESS
target: middle pectorals

Standard Technique

Take a wider than shoulder width grip on a barbell. Lower the barbell to your chest. Exhale while pushing the bar back up.

Optimized Technique

Grip the bar with a medium-wide grip as shown (Fig. 18a). Grip should be wide enough that your forearms do not quite become parallel as you lower the bar (Fig. 18b). Too narrow a grip shifts the load onto the triceps and off of the chest (Fig. 18c). Lower the bar to your sternum. In performing each rep, the bar should follow a slightly angled path from your sternum to its high point directly above your shoulders (Fig. 18d,e).

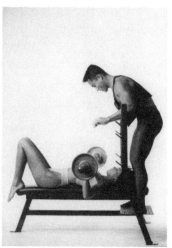

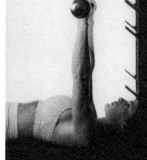

d.   e.

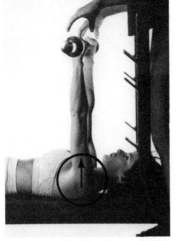

Fig. 18f—Shoulders up slightly,
off of bench

Keep your feet on the bench and your back pressed flat—don't arch. At the peak of each rep, the arms should be straight and shoulders pulled slightly up off the bench (Fig. 18f,). This is the secret to involving the entire pectoral group.

MACHINE BENCH PRESS
target: middle pectorals

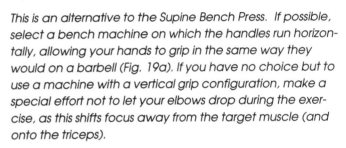

This is an alternative to the Supine Bench Press. If possible, select a bench machine on which the handles run horizontally, allowing your hands to grip in the same way they would on a barbell (Fig. 19a). If you have no choice but to use a machine with a vertical grip configuration, make a special effort not to let your elbows drop during the exercise, as this shifts focus away from the target muscle (and onto the triceps).

Adjust the bench height so that when extended, your arms will angle slightly upward. Grip the handles at a width just wider than your shoulders. At the start of the movement, elbows should angle down at about 45 degrees.

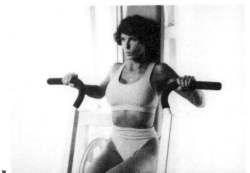
a.

Exhale as you press out, keeping your back flat against the seat (Fig. 19b). To avoid stressing the wrist joints and the risk of metacarpal tunnel syndrome, don't "break," or hyperextend, the wrists at any point.

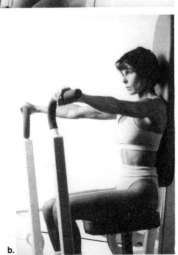
b.

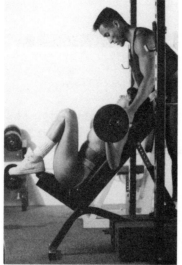

a.

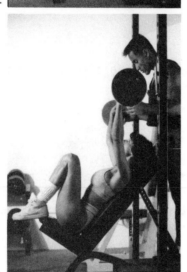

b.

INCLINE BENCH PRESS
target: upper pectorals

Because the pectoral muscles are fan-shaped, they can contract in several different directions. No single exercise can target all parts of the pectorals. This bench press variation is aimed at the <u>upper pecs</u>.

Keeping your back flat against the bench, raise the bar up and slightly back (at the peak of the movement, the bar should be more or less above your eyes) (Fig. 20a,b).

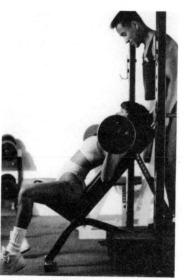

Fig. 20c—WRONG! Back arched, feet down

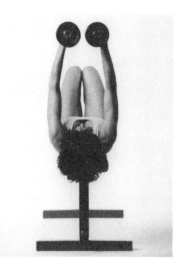

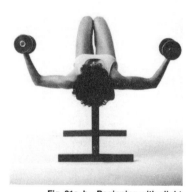

Fig. 21a, b—Beginning with slight bend in elbows; adjusting resistance by increasing bend in elbows while lowering weights (more bend, less resistance; less bend, more resistance)

PEC FLYES
target: middle pectorals

Standard Technique

Lie on your back on a bench. Holding a dumbbell in each hand, extend your arms straight up. Spread your arms to the sides. Repeat.

Optimized Technique

Lie on your back, resting your feet on the bench to prevent your back from arching during the exercise.

Holding a dumbbell in each hand, extend your arms straight up, palms facing each other. Your elbows should be slightly bent (Fig. 21a).

Spread your arms, lowering the weights to just above the level of the bench (Fig. 21b). The weights should move along a line perpendicular to your body. Feel for a stretch across your pectorals. To minimize potentially harmful strain on your biceps and elbows, bend your elbows slightly at the bottom of the motion. In the fully spread position, your palms should face up.

Moving in the largest possible arc, bring the weights together again, straightening your elbows as you go. At the peak of the motion, raise your shoulders slightly. Concentrate on feeling the effort in the muscles of your chest.

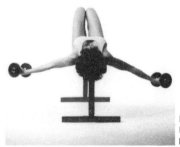

Fig. 21c—WRONG! Elbows not bent, arms below level of bench

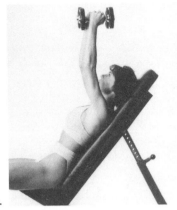

a.

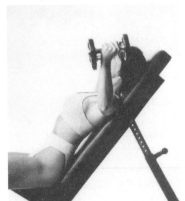

b.

INCLINE PEC FLYES
target: upper pectorals

Standard Technique

Sit on an incline bench. Holding a dumbbell in each hand, extend your arms straight up. Spread your arms and lower the weights to the sides. Reverse the motion and repeat.

Optimized Technique

The angle of the bench will determine how accurately this motion targets the upper pectorals. Set the bench to be between 30 and 45 degrees off the vertical.

In the starting position, your arms should be straight overhead, elbows slightly bent, palms facing each other (Fig. 22a,c). Spread your arms and lower the weights to approximately shoulder level, bending the elbows slightly toward the bottom of the movement to minimize joint strain. Palms should face up at this point (Fig. 22b,d). Keep your back as flat as possible.

Imagine a wall running up from the ground through both shoulders. The weights should travel along the surface of this imaginary wall.

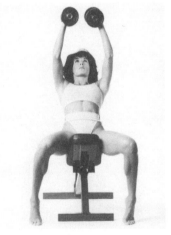

c.

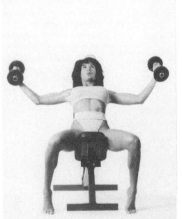

d.

Then, moving in the largest arc possible, return the weights to the starting position, straightening the elbows as you go. Press your shoulders off the bench slightly as you bring the weights together at the peak.

Concentrate on feeling the effort in the muscles of the chest.

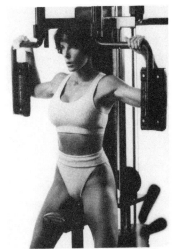

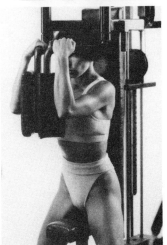

Fig. 23a, b—Swing arms in widest arc possible

PEC DECKS FLYES
target: middle pectorals.

This is essentially a machine version of Pec Flyes; some of the same points of form apply to both.

Adjust the seat height so that your upper arms are parallel to the ground (or angled up slightly; angling down can shift emphasis to the lower pecs) (Fig. 23a).

Directing the force through your elbows (not your hands), swing the pads inward (Fig. 23b). As with Pec Flys, use your shoulders to swing your arms in the <u>widest arc possible</u>. Your shoulders should be pulled forward at the peak of the movement.

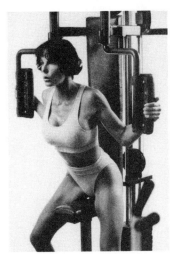

Fig. 23c—WRONG! Leaning forward, pushing with hands

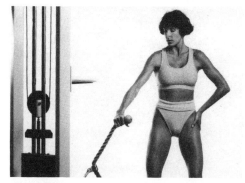

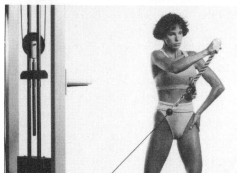

Fig. 24a, b—Pulling up and across body; maintaining constant bend in elbow

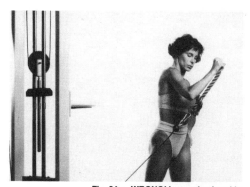

Fig. 24c—WRONG! Increasing bend in elbow while pulling arm across; twisting torso

U P P E R - P E C   C A B L E - P U L L S
target: upper pectorals

This exercise is extremely effective for isolating the upper pectorals.

Use either a rope attachment or a towel draped over the handle at the end of the cable.

Stand sideways to a low-pulley machine, about three feet away. Angle your body slightly toward the machine.

Grasp the rope or towel with the hand closest to the machine (Fig. 24a). Maintaining a constant, slight bend in your elbow, pull the rope up and diagonally across your body (Fig. 24b). Stop when your hand reaches shoulder level, or slightly above. Hold for a second, then reverse the motion. Repeat.

Two important <u>dont's</u>: *Don't increase the elbow bend as you pull, and don't twist at the waist (Fig. 24c). Either of these will shift the burden onto other muscles with better leverage, rendering the exercise useless.*

Concentrate on the tension in your upper pectorals. You can even place your free hand on your upper chest to feel the muscles contract.

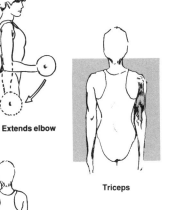

Extends shoulder

Extends elbow

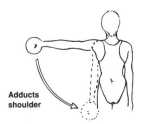

Adducts shoulder

Triceps

T R I C E P S

▲ *The **triceps** is a straight muscle composed of three seg-ments, all of which <u>extend, or straighten, the elbow</u>. In addition, one of the segments, called the **long head**, contributes to <u>shoulder adduction and extension,</u> meaning that it swings the entire arm back from the front, or pulls it toward the body from the side.*

The triceps are responsible for the shape of the back, or underside, of the upper arms.

K N E E L I N G   P U S H - U P S ,
T R I C E P S   P O S I T I O N
target: triceps

The Push-Up is a very versatile exercise and can be effec-tively made to target either the pectorals or the triceps. Push-Ups work the triceps most effectively when the el-bows are kept close to the body.

Standard Technique

Begin with fingers facing forward, hands slightly less than shoulder width apart. Lower your body to the floor keep-ing arms in against your body. Push up and repeat.

Optimized Technique

Place your hands on the ground at the level of your upper chest, rather than your shoulders. In the "up" position, they should angle slightly under you (Fig. 25a). As you lower yourself, consciously pull your arms in against your sides. This will increase the tension in the triceps (Fig. 25b).

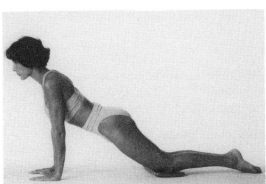

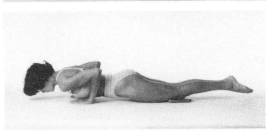

Fig. 25a,b—Arms against body to focus on the triceps

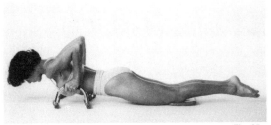

You can decrease the pressure on your wrists and increase range of motion by doing the exercise using Push-Up handles (Fig. 25c).

You can shift the emphasis of the exercise from outer to inner triceps by facing fingers out instead of forward.

Fig. 25c.

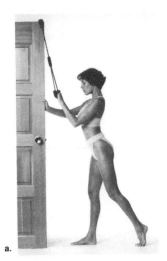

a.

b.

STRAP TRICEPS EXTENSIONS
target: triceps

Standard Technique

Secure one end of the strap, and, holding the other end, extend the elbow downward against resistance.

Optimized Technique

There are many positions in which you can accomplish the action described above; the most comfortable and the ones with minimum joint stress are as follows:

Using a Door: *Slip one end of a strap over the top of a door. Grasp the other end in your right hand, palm down (Fig. 26a). Keeping your elbow fixed by your side, extend your arm (Fig. 26b). You can increase the tension in the triceps by pulling the arm against your side as you perform the movement.*

Don't let your arm travel back or out to the side during the extension—both decrease the tension in the triceps. Letting your arm drift to the side also puts potentially injurious stress on your elbow.

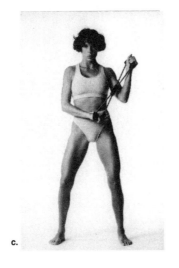

c.

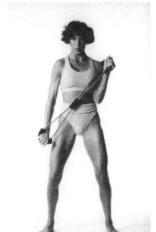

d.

Freestanding: Hold the strap as shown in Figure 26c. Flex your left shoulder up and back until your left upper arm is in line with your body and your left forearm is pointed diagonally down.

Without moving your right upper arm, extend your right elbow (Fig. 26d). You may have to experiment a bit to find the exact angle that's most comfortable. Slowly release the pressure. Repeat for 6 to 8 reps with each triceps.

You can increase the resistance by drawing the left elbow farther up and back, and by slightly flexing the left triceps to pre-stretch the strap (Fig. 26e). You can decrease it by allowing the elbow farther down and forward.

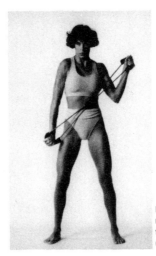

Fig. 26e—Increasing the resistance by drawing the supporting elbow up and back

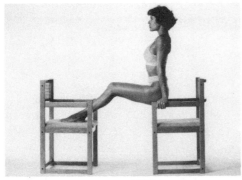

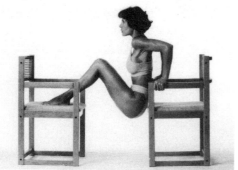

Fig. 27a, b—Keeping body upright to focus tension on the triceps

D I P S

target: triceps

Using a Chair: Make sure the arms of the chair can support your weight. If the chair were to break during the exercise, you could be injured.

Sit on the chair and elevate your feet on another chair. Grab the chair arms with palms facing in, hands beside your hips (Fig. 27a).

Sit up straight. Keeping your arms in against your sides, lower yourself (Fig. 27b). (Hunching forward shifts the emphasis off of the triceps and onto the pecs.)

Using Push-Up Handles: *Sit on the ground with legs extended, knees slightly bent. Gripping the push-up handles, palms facing in, place them onthe ground at your hips (Fig. 27c).*

Sit up straight. Supporting yourself on your heels, press yourself up keeping your arms in against your sides (Fig. 27d). Again, if you hunch over during the exercise, the emphasis shifts off of the triceps and onto the pecs.

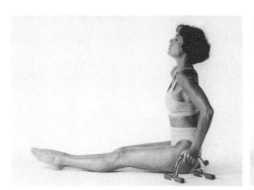

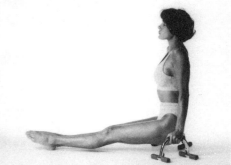

Fig. 27c, d—Using Push-Up handles to increase range of motion

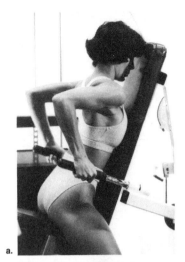

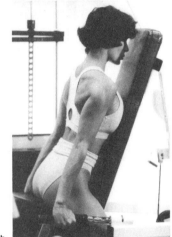

a.

b.

M A C H I N E   D I P S
target: triceps

Most dip machines are designed to work anterior delts and pectorals at the same time as triceps, somewhat diluting your triceps workout.

To Focus On the Triceps, set the dip machine arms, if adjustable, to the narrowest setting. Straddle the seat, facing into the machine. If necessary, use your legs to hold your body in place on the seat (Fig. 28a).

Grasp the handles at a point slightly behind your back and extend your arms, keeping them close to your sides. Press to full extension (Fig. 28b). Hold for a second, then return to starting position.

Note: *In case someone tells you you're using the machine "wrong," here's the explanation: The only way to focus dips on your triceps is to extend your arms at an angle slightly behind your body. This is impossible using the machine the "right" way, since most manufacturers deliberately place the handles in front of the body to involve the pectorals and the anterior deltoid.*

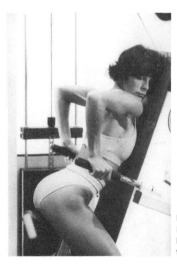

**Fig. 28c—WRONG!
Back arched;
head turned to
the side**

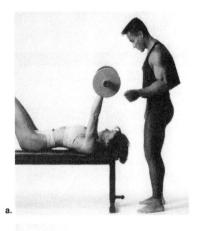

a.

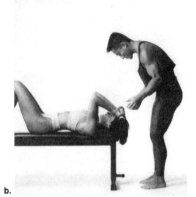

b.

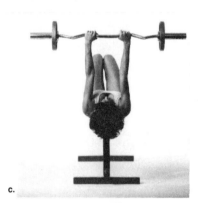

c.

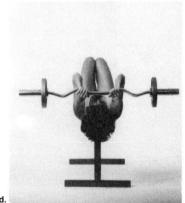

d.

LYING FRENCH PRESS
target: triceps

Standard Technique

Lie on a bench with a barbell across your thighs. Grasp the bar with a narrow, palms-down grip, elbows straight, and kick your legs up to help get the bar into position above your head. (This technique is only necessary if you are using especially heavy weights.) Keeping your upper arms stationary, bend at the elbows and lower the bar to your forehead. Press the bar back up and repeat.

Optimized Technique

Bend your knees and place your feet on the bench. This will reduce any tendency to arch your back during the movement.

At the top of each rep, your arms should be inclined back slightly toward your head (Fig. 29a,c). This angle enables you to maintain tension on the triceps between reps.

As you lower the bar to your forehead, keep your forearms parallel to each other and your upper arms stationary (Fig. 29b,d). Any deviation dilutes the exercise and strains the elbows (Fig. 29e).

This exercise lends itself well to forced reps. Have your partner slow the bar as it approaches your head, take the weight at the moment you shift direction, and then help you get it started back up. Forcing reps allows you to use heavier weights with less risk of injury.

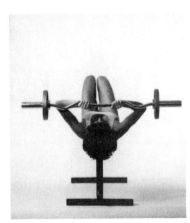

Fig. 29e—WRONG! Elbows drifting out of line

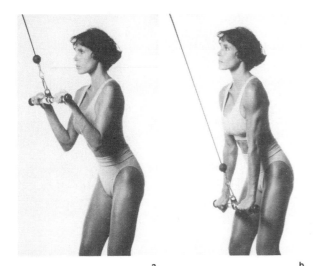

a.   b.

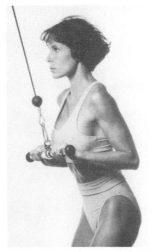

Fig. 30c—WRONG!
Elbows too
far back

TRICEPS PRESS-DOWNS
target: triceps

This exercise can be adjusted to focus on either the inner triceps (the long and medial heads) or the outer triceps (lateral head).

To focus on the inner triceps: *Use a straight or slightly bent bar at the end of a lat machine cable. Stand about 12 inches from the pulley so that the cable angles slightly away from you (Fig. 30a).*

Press the bar down in as wide an arc as possible (Fig. 30b). Don't allow your elbows to drift back (Fig. 30c). Keep your wrists straight and your shoulders down. At the bottom of the motion, allow the wrists to bend slightly back. This will help keep tension in the triceps. Don't allow your wrists to bend back more than about halfway; doing so can, in time, cause metacarpal tunnel syndrome (Fig 30d).

At the bottom of the motion, your elbows should be one or two inches in front of you, and your forearms parallel.

To focus on the outer triceps: *Drape a towel around the cable and over the bar, and grasp the ends so that your palms face each other.*

Keep your elbows fixed at a point about two inches in front of your body. Do not let them drift sideways or forward. The idea is still to describe as wide an arc as possible, without moving the elbows from their fixed positions.

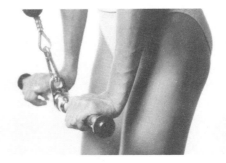

Fig. 30d—WRONG!
Wrists bent back
too far

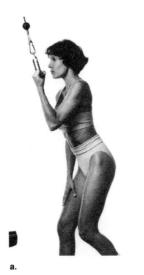
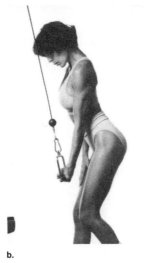

a.

b.

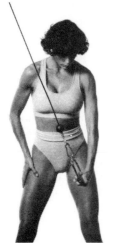
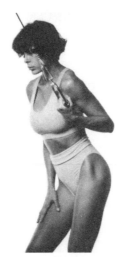

**Fig. 31c—Standing
sideways to
machine to
minimize elbow
strain**

**Fig. 31d—WRONG!
Elbow too far back**

ONE - HAND REVERSE - GRIP PRESS - DOWNS

target: outer triceps

This exercise maximizes forearm supination, focusing the effort on the triceps' lateral head.

Standard Technique

Grasp a pulley-cable handle, palm up. Keeping your elbow close to your body, extend the arm by straightening the elbow. Reverse the motion and repeat.

Optimized Technique

Use the tallest pulley machine available. Face the machine, standing about two feet from it. Take a step back with your left foot. Grasp the cable handle with your left hand, palm up. Bend both knees, and pull down so that your elbow is about six inches in front of your body (Fig 31a). The cable should travel at an angle away from you, rather than straight up.

Keeping your elbow fixed in space, extend your right arm at the elbow. Allow your wrist to bend up slightly at the bottom of the movement to maintain tension in the triceps (Fig. 31b). Your palm should remain facing up. Hold for a second, then reverse the motion.

If you experience any elbow discomfort, try standing sideways to the machine and pulling diagonally down across your body (Fig 31c).

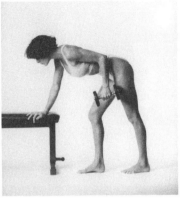

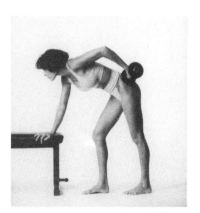

Fig. 30a, b—Keep upper arm
against side throughout
movement

TRICEPS KICK-BACKS
target: triceps

Standard Technique

Hold a light-weight dumbbell (5 to 10 lbs.) in your right hand. Lean forward so that your torso is parallel to the floor and support yourself by placing your left hand on a low bench (Fig. 32a). Bend the elbow holding the weight such that the upper arm runs along your torso, and your forearm points straight down. Straighten your elbow. Lower and repeat.

Optimized Technique

The secret of this exercise is to keep your upper arm glued to the side of your torso while you extend the elbow (Fig. 32b). If it drifts up or down, it dilutes the exercise's effectiveness (Fig. 32c,d).

Also, as you extend the elbow, rotate the wrist inward (this is called <u>pronating</u> the wrist). At full elbow extension, the palm should face the ceiling. Reverse the rotation as you lower the weight.

Make sure that your shoulder, elbow and wrist remain in line throughout the movement.

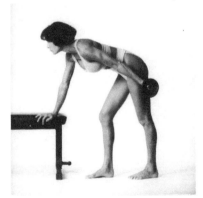

Fig. 32c—WRONG!
Elbow too high

Fig. 30d—WRONG!
Elbow too low

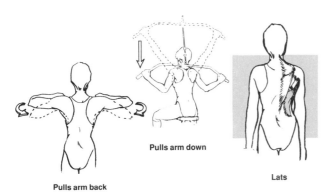

CHAPTER EIGHT

Pulls arm down

Pulls arm back

Lats

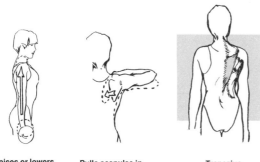

Raises or lowers shoulders

Pulls scapulae in toward spine

Trapezius

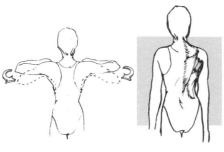

Pulls upper arm toward scapula

Teres Major, TeresMinor, Infraspinatus

UPPER BACK

▲ The **latissimus dorsi** runs from the front surface of the upper arm, underneath the shoulder, spreading out as it wraps around the sides of the torso to attach to the spine. It is responsible for <u>pulling the arm down and toward the rear,</u> as well as <u>pulling the shoulders down and rotating them inward.</u>

▲ The **trapezius** is one of four major muscles that anchor the scapulae (shoulder blades), and is responsible for the shape of the upper back where it joins the neck. The fibers spread from the shoulder to the center line, attaching along the spine from the middle back to the base of the skull. Depending on which portion of the muscle contracts, the trapezius can <u>raise or lower the shoulders,</u> or <u>pull the shoulder blades in toward the spine.</u>

▲ The **teres major**, **teres minor**, and **infraspinatus** are relatively short, straight muscles, originating along the outside edge of the scapula. The two teres muscles bracket the upper arm—the teres major attaching to the front of the humerus, and the teres minor to the rear. Alternately, they contribute to <u>inward and outward rotation of the arm.</u> All three muscles <u>pull the upper arm toward the scapula.</u>

Functionally, all the upper-back muscles work together. They contract along a number of lines, ranging from straight across the back to nearly up-and-down. A good back routine should involve contractions along as many lines as possible between these extremes.

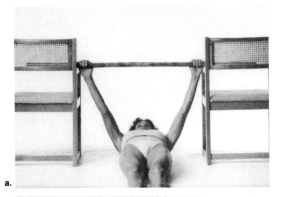

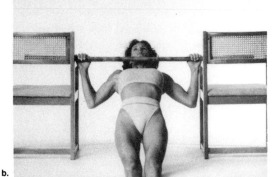

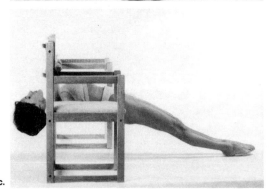

Fig. 33—Doing Supine Pull-Ups with a wide grip targets the upper lats and center traps

SUPINE PULL-UPS
target: latissimus dorsi, teres major & minor, center and/or lower trapezius

This exercise uses a bar about 24 inches off the ground. Unless your gym has a low bar, you can use two chairs and a stout pole—a heavy broom handle works well. **Warning: Make sure the chairs are stable and that the broom handle is strong enough to take your weight. You could be severely injured if the pole were to break or the chairs to slip.**

Standard Technique

Lie on your back beneath a low bar. Grasp the bar with a wide, overhand grip. Pull up until your chest touches the bar.

Lower and repeat for 6 to 8 reps.

Optimized Technique

This exercise can be modified to focus on the lower lats/lower traps or on the upper lats/center traps.

To focus on upper lats/center traps: Grasp the bar with a <u>wide overhand grip</u> (Fig. 33a). Pull up so the bar touches your <u>upper chest</u> (Fig. 33b,c). Hold for a second at the peak, then lower slowly and repeat.

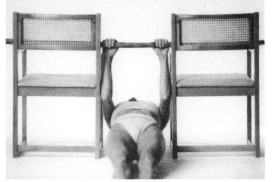

Fig. 33d—Supine Pull-Ups with a
narrow grip focuses on the lower lats
and lower traps

To focus on lower lats/lower traps: *Grasp the bar with a shoulder-width grip (Fig. 33d) and pull up to the bar. Hold for a second at the peak, then lower slowly and repeat.*

STRAP SEATED ROWS
target: latissimus dorsi, teres major & minor, lower trapezius

Warning: Be very careful when using any kind of elastic strap that it doesn't slip loose and hit you on the body or in the face. You could be severely injured if this happens. Never place your face in line with a stretched band.

Standard Technique

Sit on the floor with legs together, knees bent. Anchor the midpoint of the strap around your arches. Grasp the strap ends, palms in, and extend your knees until they are nearly straight. Pull back. Hold for a second, then release slowly and repeat. **Make sure the strap is positioned so it doesn't slip off your feet while you're doing the exercise.**

Optimized Technique

To focus on lower lats/lower traps: (Low Position): *Grab the strap ends, palms down, arms extended as far as possible (Fig. 34a). Feel for the stretch across your middle back.*

Pull back on the handles, bringing your elbows toward your waist and gradually rotating your forearms outward. Your palms should finish facing up (Fig. 34b). Try to have the feeling of pulling your elbows back and down. Con-

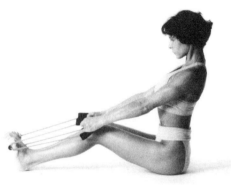

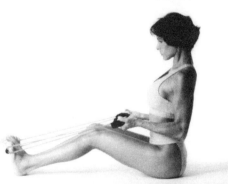

Fig. 34a,b— Bringing elbows down to the
waist to focus on lower lats / traps

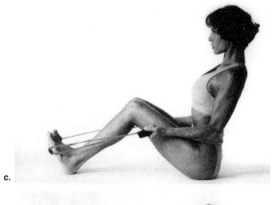

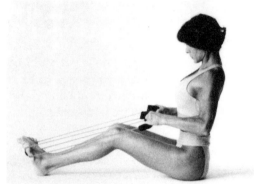

c.

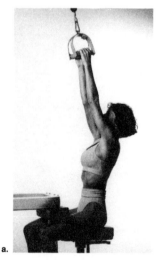

a.

centrate on feeling the effort in your back, not your biceps. Slowly release and repeat.

Resistance can be adjusted by varying the bend in your knees (Fig. 34c).

To focus on upper lats/center traps: (High Position): *From the same starting position, pull back on the handles bring-ing your elbows out to the sides. Your elbows should finish halfway between shoulder and waist level (Fig. 34d). (Any higher will shift the focus to the rear delts, decreasing the exercise's effectiveness.)*

Palms should remain down throughout the movement. As before, try not to flex your biceps. Again, resistance will vary with the angle of your knees—experiment until it feels comfortable.

Slowly release and repeat.

Fig. 34d—Bringing elbows up to focus on upper lats / mid traps

C L O S E - G R I P   P U L L - D O W N S
target: latissimus dorsi, teres major & minor, center & lower trapezius

Standard Technique

Facing the lat machine, sit as close as possible to the restraining bar. Grasp the V-grip with your thumbs at the narrow end.

Pull down to your chest, arching your back and thrusting your chest up to meet the bar. Slowly release.

Optimized Technique

Start in the position described above, but in addition, lean back <u>slightly</u> so that your shoulders are raised and your lats stretched as much as possible (Fig. 35a). Beginning the ex-

ercise in this "pre-stretched" position ensures that all sections of the muscle can contract through their full range.

In pulling down, bring the bar to your <u>lower chest</u>, rather than your upper chest. As you do so, arch your back and thrust your chest up to meet the bar, while simultaneously leaning farther and farther back until, by the end of the movement, your torso is about 3/4 of the way to being parallel to the floor (Fig. 35b).

Slowly release, and return to a nearly upright position, shoulders extended, maintaining the lat stretch you had before the rep.

Note: Don't hunch forward during the exercise (Fig. 35c). Hunching turns the exercise into an undesirable sit-up-like motion that brings the abdominals into play and increases the contribution of the biceps at the expense of the lats. Keeping the back arched assures maximum lat involvement.

The key to this exercise—and all upper-back exercises—is to pull from your back, rather than your arms. The Pull-Down should begin with <u>shoulder movement</u>, not elbow flexion. The shoulders should move back and down with the shoulder blades pulling toward each other—only then should the elbows begin to bend. It should feel as though the motion originates at the bottom of your lats (i.e., in a contraction drawing your shoulders to your spine.)

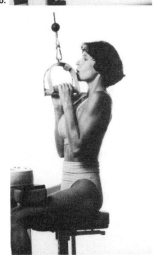

b.

Fig. 35—WRONG!
Upright body
decreases lat
involvement

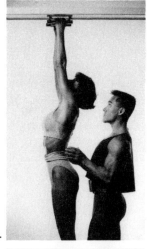

a.

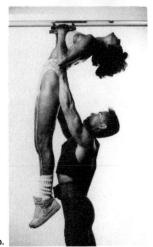

b.

Fig. 36

C L O S E - G R I P   P U L L - U P S
target: latissimus dorsi, teres major & minor, center & loser trapezius

Close-Grip Pull-Ups are the bodyweight equivalent of Close-Grip Pull-Downs. Both exercises target the same muscle groups and involve motions that are almost identical. Similar points of form apply to both.

Standard Technique

This very advanced exercise requires a horizontal bar (i.e., a chinning bar) and an inverted V handle. Grasp the V and pull yourself up, aiming to touch your chest to the bar. Lower slowly and repeat.

Optimized Technique

Grasp the handle and hang with your shoulders extended as far as possible. Feel the stretch in your lats (Fig. 36a).Tilt your head back, arch your chest and slowly pull up, aiming to touch your sternum—or, if possible, your abdomen—to the bar. If the exercise feels too difficult at first, have a partner support part of your weight as you lift (Fig. 36b).

It's very important to maintain an extreme backward arch throughout the movement. The temptation will be to hunch forward as the motion becomes difficult; this takes stress off the muscles you're trying to work. Better to go up only a few inches with correct form.

Lower slowly until you are hanging again with your arms completely straight and shoulders extended.

This exercise works well with forced reps: Have your partner stand behind you and give you just enough help to complete the motion <u>in good form</u> by pushing up gently with both hands on your middle back.

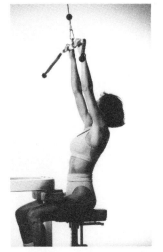

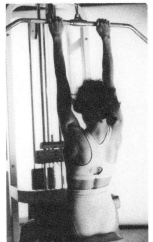

Fig. 37a, b—Shoulders
fully extended to start
(side and rear views)

SCAPULAR ROLLS
target: lats, teres major & minor, center traps

Because Close-Grip Pull-Downs (described above) involve the biceps as well as the lats, it is possible for tired biceps to limit their effectiveness as a lat exercise. Scapular Rolls, however, have little biceps component. Sets of Scapular Rolls should be interspersed with sets of Pull-Downs to help accelerate the exhaustion of the lats relative to the biceps.

Facing the lat machine, sit as close as possible to the restraining bar. Using a straight bar this time, place your hands shoulder width apart, palms away from you. Lean back slightly, allowing your shoulders to extend until you feel the stretch in your lats (Fig. 37a,b).

Concentrate on the movement of your shoulders as you pull the bar down about 6 to 12 inches. Feel the contraction of your lats along both sides of your ribcage. Your scapulae (shoulder blades) should move down and toward the center line. Elbows should bend only slightly (Fig. 37c,d).

Hold for a second, then slowly release, feeling again the stretch in the lats as your shoulders rise. This is a subtle, small-range motion that may take some practice.

Note: *Scapular Rolls are only intended for use with a biceps-dependent upper-back exercise like Close-Grip Pull-Downs. They are not effective used by themselves.*

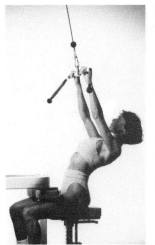 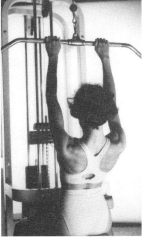

Fig. 37c,d—Shoulder blades moving down and back; very
little bend in the elbows

HFL DECLINE ROWS
target: lats, center & lower traps, teres major & minor, infraspinatus

This exercise allows you to use relatively heavy weights for the sake of efficiency while minimizing the stress on your lower back.

Adjust an incline bench to an angle of about 30 to 40 degrees. If your gym doesn't have an adjustable incline bench, you can use a flat bench with one end elevated on a block. Make certain the bench is stable before beginning the exercise!

Lean over the high end of the bench, supporting yourself on your abdominals. Your arms should hang naturally off the bench, with the dumbbells slightly forward and held at an angle of about 45 degrees to the center line of the bench. Bend your elbows slightly and allow the shoulders to extend fully. You should feel a stretch across your middle back and in your lats (Fig. 38a).

Concentrate on starting the lift with a movement of your scapulae together. As you pull, raise your chest slightly but keep your abdominals in firm contact with the bench to reduce pressure on the lower back. Keeping your elbows close to your sides, lift until they reach waist level. Rotate your wrists as you lift so that your palms end up facing one another (Fig. 38b).

It's important to think of lifting <u>back</u> and not just up. Your forearms and biceps should be as relaxed as possible (except for the effort of gripping the dumbbell). Feel for the tension in your lower lats and center back.

Reverse the motion to lower the weights. The dumbbells should end up not quite as far forward as they started, and not touching the ground. As you lower the weight, reverse the rotation of your wrists so that the dumbbells return to their initial 45-degree angle to the bench. Keep your elbows bent to get the maximum stretch across the center back and lower lats.

Remember to lean against the bench throughout the exercise to keep the strain off your lower back.

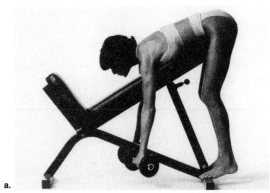

a.

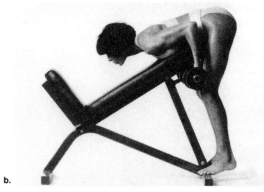

b.

Fig. 38

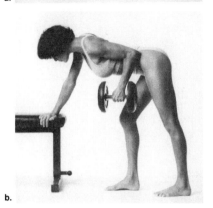
a.

b.

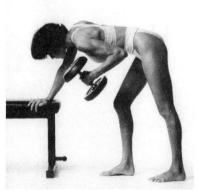

Fig. 39c—WRONG! Arm not relaxed;
triceps flexed

Fig. 39d—WRONG! Arm not relaxed;
biceps flexed

STANDING ONE-HAND ROWS

target: lats, center & lower traps, teres major & minor, infraspinatus

One-Hand Rows can be used instead of HFL Decline Rows if no decline bench is available.

Standard Technique

Stand with left foot forward, right foot back, knees bent. Bend over until your torso is roughly parallel to the floor, and place your left hand on a bench or chair for support. Your right arm (holding the weight) should be extended straight toward the floor.

Lift the weight straight up toward your shoulder. Hold for a second at the peak, then slowly lower.

Optimized Technique

The two most important factors in any rowing exercise are (1) the feeling that the lift is coming from the lats and traps, not the shoulders and arms, and (2) a full range of motion. At the bottom of the row, you must feel a stretch in the lats, and the shoulder blades must be pulled away from the spine as much as possible.

To improve focus and maximize the lat stretch:

Begin with one foot about 12 inches ahead of the other. Bend your knees slightly (Fig. 39a).

Lift the weight until your upper arm and elbow reach the level of your back (Fig. 39b). Keep your upper arm relaxed and the elbow joint loose: the weight should hang naturally from your elbow (Fig. 39c,d).

Note: *Many people lift their elbows higher, believing this will maximize center trap involvement (Fig. 39e). It won't— at least, not necessarily. The center traps function only to pull your shoulder blades toward the spine. The best way to maximize their involvement is to raise the arm until the elbow is even with the body, then concentrate on pulling the shoulder blades together.*

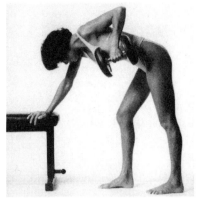

Hold for a second at the top of the movement, then lower the weight down across your body so it ends up between your feet. Feel for a stretch in your lats. Alternate sets with each arm.

Fig. 39e—WRONG! Elbow too high

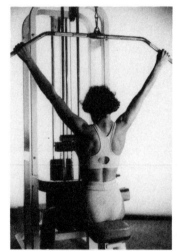

Fig. 40a—Grip wide enough so forearms are never parallel during exercise

WIDE-GRIP PULL-DOWNS

target: latissimus dorsi

Standard Technique

Using a wide grip, pull down on the lat bar until it touches the back of your neck. Release and repeat.

Optimized Technique

Spread your grip on the bar wide enough that your forearms are never parallel during the movement (Fig. 40a). As you pull down, pull out and back as well (Fig. 40b,c). You shouldn't have to drop your head forward or hunch over to allow the bar to pass behind your head (Fig. 40d).

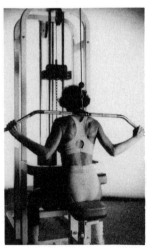

b.

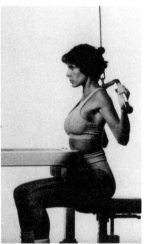

c.

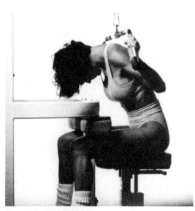

Fig. 40d.—WRONG! Keep body upright and head forward throughout exercise

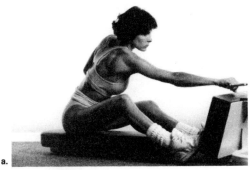

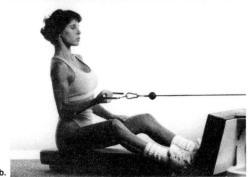

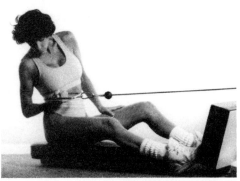

Fig. 41c—WRONG! Elbow should not cross behind line of body

SEATED ONE-HAND ROWS
target: lower lats, center traps

One-handed rowing allows the use of lighter weights than two-handed rowing, sparing your lower back unnecessary stress. It also allows the greatest possible lat stretch in the extended position, increasing the exercise's range of motion. Finally, when performed as indicated, Seated One-Hand Rows concentrate on the hard-to-develop lower lats.

Standard Technique

Sit with legs extended, braced against the seated rowing bar. Grasp the cable handle with one hand, extending your arm forward. Pull straight back, twisting your body until your elbow is as far back as possible. Slowly release.

Optimized Technique

Sit with legs extended, <u>knees bent</u>, feet braced against the seated rowing bar. (Straight legs increase the chance of injury caused by limitations in hamstring and lower-back flexibility.)

Lean forward, arm (and <u>shoulder</u>) extended straight in front of you, palm down, gripping the handle (Fig. 41a). If the cable is slack in this position, use a box beneath your feet to position yourself farther from the machine.

As you pull back, rotate your wrist outward about 150 degrees so that your palm finishes facing up. At the same time, straighten your torso and thrust your chest forward. You should finish in a <u>slightly</u> backward-leaning posture (Fig. 41b). (Leaning back too far dilutes the effectiveness of the exercise; this is a common error.)

As in standing One-Hand Rows, the elbow should not cross behind the line of your body (Fig. 41c). Once your elbow reaches your side, concentrate on bringing the shoulder back and the shoulder blade toward the spine.

Reverse the motion, remembering to reverse the rotation of your wrist. Finish with your shoulder extended as far as possible.

CHAPTER NINE

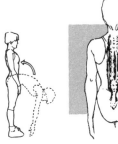

Straighten back   **Spinal Erectors**

LOWER BACK

▲ *The **spinal erectors** are a group of muscle segments that run vertically along the spine, linking various points along the lumbar, thoracic, and cervical vertebrae. Together, they <u>extend, or straighten, the back</u>.*

Because of their role in maintaining good posture, strong spinal erectors are particularly important for optimum health.

*At advanced levels of **Transfigure II**, the spinal erectors get a good workout just from serving as stabilizers in other exercises. However, the muscle group is so important in promoting general health (as well as preventing spinal injuries) that you should include targeted spinal erector work in your routine as well.*

HYPEREXTENSIONS
target: spinal erectors

Hyperextensions are best done on a bench made for the purpose, but can, in a pinch, be done on the edge of a resilient surface like a padded table, arm of a sofa, or the like, with someone holding your ankles.

Standard Technique

Hang from the waist, facedown, over the edge of the bench. Lightly rest your hands behind your head or neck. Slowly straighten your body to a horizontal position. Hold for a second, then lower and repeat.

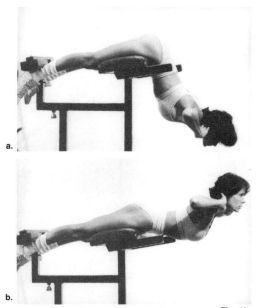

a.

b.

Fig. 42

Optimized Technique

Begin as described above (Fig. 42a). Throughout the exercise, hold your head as far back as possible and arch your back, as in a swan dive. <u>Maintain this arch even at the bottom of the movement</u>. Make the lifting motion slow and smooth; don't use momentum to lift yourself. Raise yourself to a point slightly above the horizontal (Fig. 42b).

***Note:** Don't try to lace your fingers behind your head, as this will limit your ability to arch backward.*

CHAPTER TEN

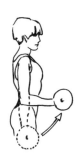

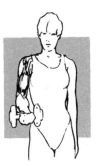

**Flexes
shoulder**

**Bends
elbow**

**Biceps,
Long Head**

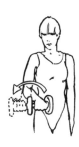

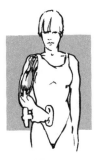

**Supinates
forearm**

**Biceps,
Short Head**

BICEPS

*The **biceps** is a straight muscle composed of two segments, or heads, each of which has its own function.*

▲ *The **long head** of the biceps runs from the shoulder to
the forearm. It <u>bends the elbow</u> and <u>raises the arm forward at the shoulder</u>.*

▲ *The **short head** of the biceps also runs from shoulder to
forearm—but at a different angle, allowing it to
<u>supinate the forearm</u> (rotate it outward).*

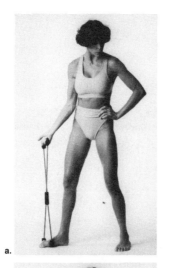

a.

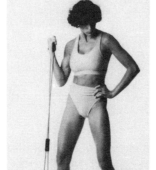

b.

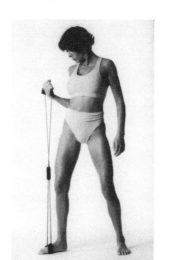

Fig. 43c—WRONG!
Elbow too far back

S T R A P   C U R L S
target: biceps, emphasis on the long head

Standard Technique

Anchor one end of the strap around your foot and grip the other end, palm up. Curl toward your shoulder. Hold for a moment, then lower and repeat. Alternate sets for each arm.

Optimum Technique

Step forward with your right foot and anchor one end of the strap around it. Grip the other end with your right hand, palm up (Fig. 43a). (Pulling at this angle matches the strap's resistance to the biceps' force more effectively than pulling straight up.)

Curl toward your shoulder, allowing your elbow to travel forward about four inches over the course of the lift (Fig. 43b). Don't let your elbow drift to the side—this can strain the joint. If necessary, support the pulling arm against the back of your other hand, just to learn the motion. Lower and repeat. Don't let your elbow drift behind the line of your body (Fig 43c).

To Make It Harder: *You can increase resistance two ways: first, by stepping farther forward with the front foot, and second, by bending your wrist back slightly at the peak of the movement. (Be careful not to bend all the way back, as this can, in time, damage the wrist.)*

To Make It Easier: *Decrease resistance by placing your front foot on a block. The taller the block, the lower the resistance.*

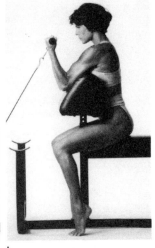

a.

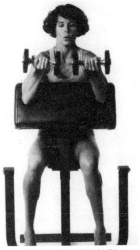

b.

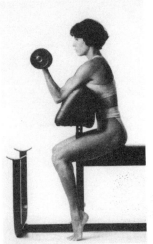

Fig. 44c—Preacher curls
with dumbbells;
curl both arms at
the same time

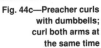

Fig. 44d—WRONG! Elbows
out of line with
shoulders and
hands

PREACHER CURLS
target: biceps

Preacher Curls have two advantages over the Standing Barbell Curl: (1) They put much less strain on the lower back, and (2) they do a better job of isolating the biceps.

Standard Technique

This exercise can be done with a standard barbell, with dumbbells, or with a straight or angled bar attached to a low-pulley machine.

Take a shoulder-width grip on the bar. Position yourself with the bench under your armpits. Curl the weight to your chin, keeping your upper arms parallel throughout the motion. Lower and repeat.

Optimized Technique

If you have a low-pulley machine available (ideally one with an angled bar), we recommend using it. The pulley offers better resistance than the free weights; the angled bar puts the least possible strain on the wrists.

Take a slightly <u>less</u> than shoulder-width grip on the bar; this will reduce stress on the elbows. Position yourself so that the bench supports you about mid-chest, or a bit lower. Approximately the lower <u>half</u> of your upper arms should be in contact with the bench. Lean slightly over the bench (Fig. 44a).

Curl the bar to your chin, leaning into the movement (Fig. 44b). This will help maintain a constant tension in the biceps. Reverse the motion and repeat.

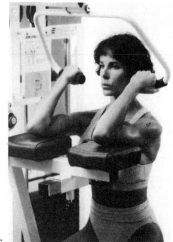

Fig. 45a—Seat adjusted
so arms are parallel
with floor

b.

MACHINE BICEPS CURLS
target: biceps

Adjust the seat height so that your upper arms are parallel to the floor (Fig. 45a). As you curl, keep your wrists straight. Your elbows should remain pointing forward; allowing them to drift to the sides can place potentially damaging stress on the joints. Curl as far as possible; at the peak of the motion, there should be some sensation of your upper arm lifting, as though you were trying to reach over your shoulders (Fig. 45b).

Do not elevate the shoulders or hunch forward at the peak of the motion (Fig. 45c).

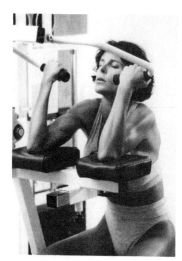

**Fig. 45c—WRONG!
Don't elevate
shoulders or
hunch forward**

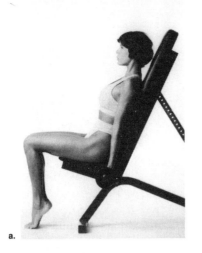

a.

SEATED DUMBBELL CURLS
target: biceps

Curl until your arms are almost vertical (Fig. 46a,b). At this point, you can rock your wrists back <u>slightly</u> to increase resistance on the biceps (Fig. 46c). Reverse the motion and repeat.

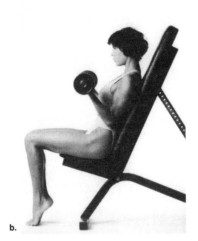

b.

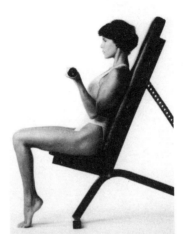

Fig. 46c—Wrist rocked back slightly

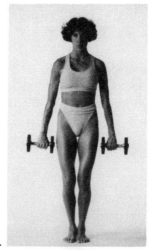

a.

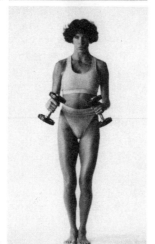

b.

STANDING SUPINATED DUMBBELL CURLS
target: biceps, brachialis

As one of the functions of the biceps is to supinate (rotate outward) the hand, a complete biceps workout must employ dumbbells, since, clearly, it's impossible to supinate when both hands are gripping the same bar. The points discussed here apply to all supinated curls, standing or seated.

Standard Technique

Begin with a dumbbell in each hand, arms at your sides, palms facing back (Fig. 47a). Curl both arms forward, rotating them outward as you do. At the peak of the motion, your palms should face up (Fig. 47b,c,d). Lower, reversing the rotation, and repeat with the other arm. Repeat continuing to alternate arms.

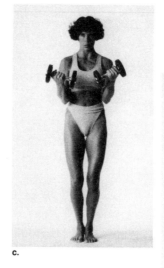

c.

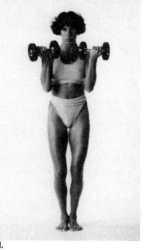

d.

Optimized Technique

Begin as described above. (You can increase your stability, and decrease general strain by leaning against a bench with knees slightly bent.)

Think of the exercise as consisting of two simultaneous movements that must blend smoothly:

▲ *Supination of the forearms. This is simply a 180 degree rotation of the forearms, from palms down to palms up.*

▲ *A proper curl. This requires concentration, since, left alone, the body will generally adjust itself to the position of greatest mechanical advantage, thereby doing as little work as possible.*

To achieve an effective curl...

▲ *Make sure the weights travel upward exactly in line with the direction you're facing. Shoulder, elbow, and hand should all remain on this line.*

▲ *Keep your elbows slightly in front of your body. Letting them drift back to your side, or worse, behind your body, takes strain off the target muscles (Fig. 47e,f). Lean slightly into the curl at the top to keep tension in the muscle.*

These two actions, supination and curling, should both begin and end at the same time. (A common error is to perform the entire supination at the outset.) It's important to exactly reverse the motion on the way down. Don't let elbows or arms drift from their position.

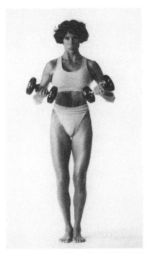

Fig. 47e—WRONG!
Elbows not in line with
shoulders and hands

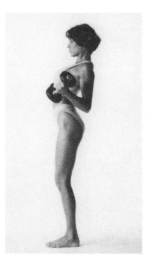

Fig. 47f—WRONG!
Elbows too far back

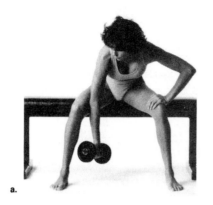

a.

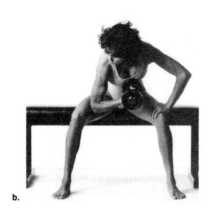

b.

SEATED SUPINATED DUMBBELL CURLS

target: biceps, brachialis

This exercise works the target muscles from a different angle than the exercises described above, and is a good complement to those exercises.

Sit at the edge of the bench with your legs apart. Rest your right elbow against the inside of your right thigh. Hold a dumbbell in your right hand, palm down to start (Fig. 48a). Curl the weight toward your right shoulder, rotating your forearm outward as you go. At the peak, your palm should face up (Fig. 48b). Lower the weight, reversing the rotation, and repeat. Alternate sets using each arm.

Here, as in the standing curl described above, supination of the forearm must be smoothly integrated with the curl. And here again, the elbow, shoulder, and hand must remain in line with each other throughout. Don't let the elbow move in toward the groin; this lowers the resistance on the biceps and may strain the elbow (Fig 48c).

Do not lean back to cheat the weight up (Fig 48d). Doing so defeats the exercise. If you need help to make it through your reps, push from below with the supporting leg, or use your other hand to provide forced reps.

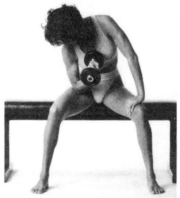

**Fig. 48c—WRONG!
Elbow moving in
toward groin**

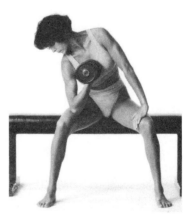

**Fig. 48d—WRONG!
Leaning back**

CHAPTER ELEVEN

DELTOIDS

*The **deltoids** are a group of three fan-shaped muscle segments running from the collar bone to the upper arm.*

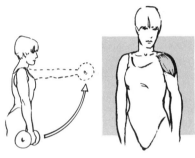

Raises arm forward   **Front Delt**

▲ *The **anterior**, or front, deltoid <u>raises the arm toward the front and rotates it inward</u>.*

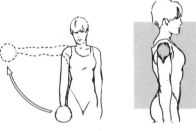

Raises arm to the side   **Side Delt**

▲ *The **lateral**, or side, deltoid <u>raises the arm to the side</u>.*

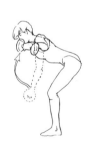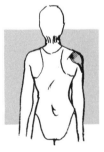

Raises arm to the rear
Rotates arm outward   **Rear Delt**

▲ *The **posterior**, or rear, deltoid <u>raises the arm toward the rear and rotates it outward</u>.*

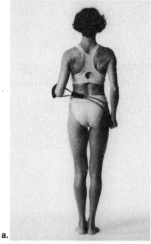

a.

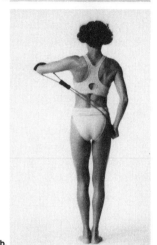

b.

Fig. 49

STRAP
SIDE DELT RAISES
target: lateral deltoid (side shoulder)

Slide the middle handle on the strap toward one end to create one large loop and one small one. Place the small loop over your left arm, just below the elbow. Pass the other end of the strap behind your back, and hold it firmly pressed against your right hip (Fig. 49a).

Maintaining a 90-degree bend in your left elbow, raise that arm sideways to the level of your shoulder. Keep your shoulder down as you lift (Fig. 49b). (Raising the shoulder shifts emphasis onto your upper traps decreasing the effectiveness of the exercise.)

Lower and repeat. Alternate sets for each arm.

***To make it harder:** Secure the strap beneath the heel of the foot opposite the lifting arm.*

***Note:** The standard form of this exercise, not described here, involves gripping the strap in the <u>hand</u> of the lifting arm, and lifting with a <u>straight</u> arm. This form places unnecessary strain on the elbow joint—we strongly recommend against it.*

STRAP
FRONT DELT RAISES
target: anterior deltoid (front shoulder)

Standard Technique

With your left arm behind your back, hold the strap with both hands facing palm down. Raise the strap forward to shoulder height. Lower and repeat.

Optimized Technique

Again, the standard form of this exercise, as described above, puts potentially injurious stress on your elbow. Use the form explained below.

Slide the middle handle on the strap toward one end to create one large loop and one small one. Place the small loop over your left arm, just below the elbow. Pass the other end of the strap behind your back and hold it at waist level with your right hand.

Fully bend the left elbow in preparation for the movement. The strap handle should cross the front of your forearm just above the elbow (Fig. 50a).

Maintaining a full bend at the elbow, sweep the elbow forward in a wide arc to shoulder level (Fig. 50b). (Don't raise your shoulder, or let the arm drift to the side—either will shift the emphasis off-target.)

Lower and repeat. Alternate sets for each arm.

To make it harder: *Secure the fixed end of the strap under the heel of the foot beneath the moving arm.*

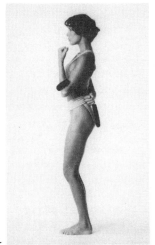

a.

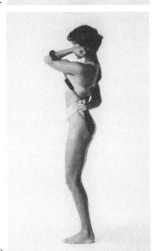

b.

Fig. 50

BOW-AND-ARROW
(Rear Deltoid)
target: posterior deltoid (rear shoulder)

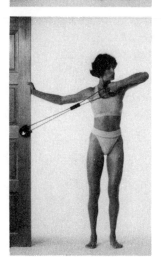

Secure one end of a strap to a door knob or any solid, immovable support at waist level. (If you have a floor plan that would allow you to do the exercise off the end of a <u>closed</u> door, this is preferable to using an open door.)

Stand sideways to the edge of the door, holding the other end of the strap in the hand farthest from the door knob. Bring the hand and arm holding the strap up to shoulder level, allowing the arm to come forward and the elbow to bend. Hold the strap palm down (Fig. 51a).

Allowing your elbow to bend freely, move the elbow straight out to side at shoulder level until your upper arm comes in line with your body and the door (Fig. 51b).

To keep the strap from slipping off the door knob, make sure that, at the peak of the movement, the strap is parallel to the door, not angled away from it. To be safe, keep your head turned away from the door during the exercise. Never place your face in line with a stretched elastic band.

Release slowly and repeat. Alternate sets with each arm.

Freestanding: *You can also do this exercise holding the fixed end of the strap with your extended arm (Fig. 51 c,d). This is less effective, since the resistance is determined by the length of your arm and can't be adjusted.*

Fig. 51a,b—Elbow moving
straight to the side
at shoulder level;
strap parallel with
front of door

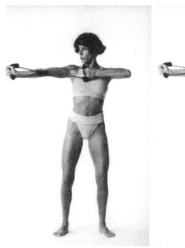

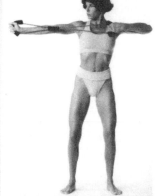

c.   d.

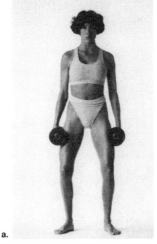

a.

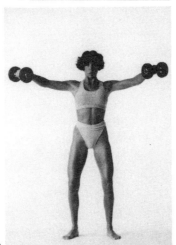

b.

DUMBBELL SIDE DELT RAISES
target: lateral deltoid (side shoulder)

Hold a pair of dumbbells at your side, palms facing in (Fig. 52a). Lift the weights up and to the side to about shoulder level (Fig. 52b). Lower and repeat.

The technique of "pouring water" (Fig. 52c), once thought to heighten the focus on the lateral deltoid, is <u>not</u> recommended because of the stress it places on the shoulder joint.

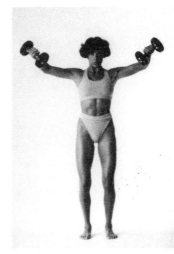

Fig. 52c—WRONG!
"Pouring water" (tipping the front ends of the dumbbells down at the peak of the movement) stresses shoulder joint

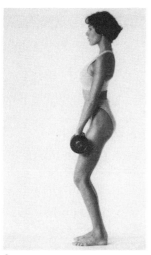
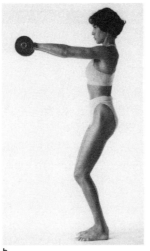

a.   b.

D U M B B E L L
F R O N T   D E L T   R A I S E S
target: anterior deltoid (front shoulder)

Hold a pair of dumbbells at your side, palms facing back (Fig. 53a). Lift the weights in front of you, keeping arms parallel, to about shoulder level (Fig. 53b). Lower and repeat.

D U M B B E L L
R E A R   D E L T   R A I S E S
target: posterior deltoid (rear shoulder)

Holding a dumbbell in each hand, bend forward at the waist until your body is nearly parallel to the floor (Fig. 54a). Your arms should hang straight down from your shoulders. Raise the weights to the side, up to body level (Fig. 54b). The weights should end up straight out from your shoulders, not back by your waist (Fig. 54c). Lower and repeat.

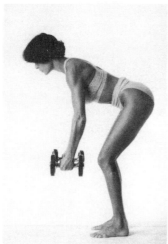
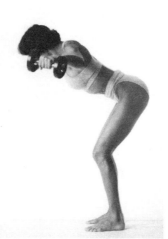
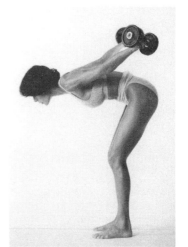

a.   b.

Fig. 54c—WRONG! Raising weights too far back

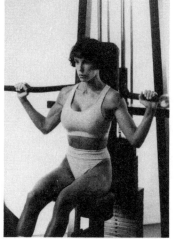

BEHIND-THE-NECK PRESS
target: lateral and anterior deltoid

Adjust the machine's seat so that the bar is at shoulder level. Grasp the handles with a wide grip (Fig. 55a). (Too narrow a grip shifts focus to the triceps; Fig. 55c.) Slowly press the bar up (Fig. 55b). Lower and repeat.

Keep your back flat against the machine seat throughout the exercise. You can injure your lower back if you arch.

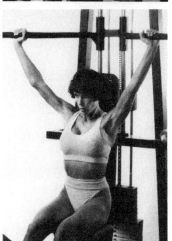

Fig. 55a,b—Keep
back flat against
seat throughout
exercise

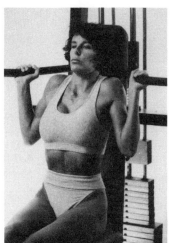

Fig. 55b—WRONG! Back arched;
shoulders hunched

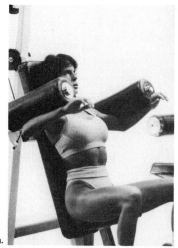

a.

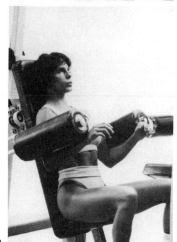

b.

MACHINE SIDE DELT RAISES
target: lateral deltoid (side shoulder)

This is a machine alternative to Strap and Dumbbell Side Delt Raises. The advantage of the machine over the free weight version of Delt Raises is that the machine eliminates any rotational stress on the elbows. Its disadvantage is that, even on the better machines, the movement feels slightly less "natural."

Adjust the seat so that your shoulders are just below the level of the arm pivots. If the seat isn't adjustable, stand with your knees bent to achieve the appropriate height.

Bend your elbows and bring the sides of your arms up against the pads (Fig. 56a). Press the pads up, just past shoulder level. Keep your back flat against the seat back throughout (Fig. 56b). Lower and repeat.

Be sure to press with your upper arms only, not your forearms. Pressing with the forearms strains the shoulder external rotators—muscles that can't handle the amount of weight appropriate to a lateral delt exercise (Fig. 56c).

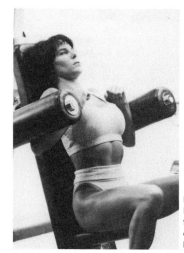

**Fig. 56c—WRONG!
Pushing up with
forearms instead
of upper arms;
back arched**

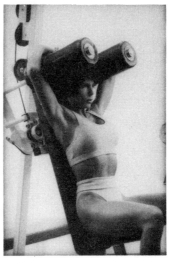

a.

MACHINE FRONT DELT RAISES
target: anterior deltoid (front shoulder)

This is a machine alternative to Strap Front Delt Raises. Again, adjust the seat so that your shoulders are just below the level of the arm pivots. If the seat isn't adjustable, stand with knees bent to reach the appropriate height.

Open your arms outward and rest the pads in the bend of your elbows (Fig. 57a). Press the pads up above head level, maintaining the bend in your elbows (Fig. 57b). Lower and repeat.

b.

FIVE-MINUTE STRETCH ROUTINE

*Here is a fast and effective stretching routine to help you remain flexible while doing the **Transfigure II** routines. These stretches have been selected and modified to maximize leverage and isolation, while minimizing joint stress.*

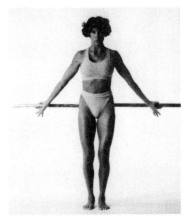

a.

b.

CHEST/FRONT SHOULDER STRETCH
target: pectorals, anterior deltoid

In a standing position, grip a five- or six-foot pole near the ends, palms down (Fig. 58a). (It isn't necessary to make fists; a loose thumb/index finger grip is better—it will allow the pole to rotate during the exercise, putting less stress on the joints.)

Keeping your arms locked at the elbows, bring the pole over your head (Fig. 58b). Move through the range where you feel the stretch and stop just beyond it. Reverse the motion, stopping above the stretch range (Fig 58c). Repeat for 4 reps. Try narrowing your grip slightly between reps to increase the intensity of the stretch on each rep.

c.

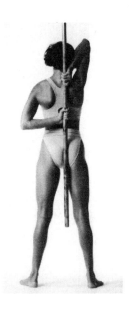

T R I C E P S   S T R E T C H
target: triceps

Hold a pole in your right hand and lower it behind you as if to scratch your back. Grasp the pole with your left hand at the level of your waist, palm facing out (Fig 59).

Pull down with your left hand and push back gently with your head. Keep your right arm as relaxed as possible. You should feel the stretch along the back of your right arm. Hold your maximum stretch for about 10 seconds, then relax. Repeat with arms reversed

L A T   S T R E T C H
target: lats

Grasping your partner's hands (or any fixed bar at about waist level), bend at the knees and waist, sinking down and backward. Feel the stretch along the sides of your torso (Fig. 60). Hold at maximum stretch for 10 seconds, then slowly straighten and relax.

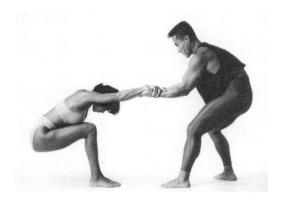

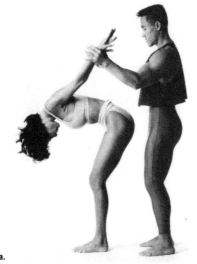

a.

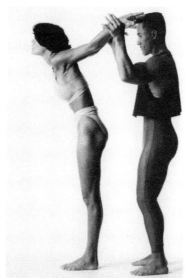

b.

BICEPS/FRONT SHOULDER STRETCH

target: biceps, anterior deltoid head

Stand facing away from your partner. Bend at the knees and the waist. Extend your arms behind you, palms facing each other. Have your partner reach beneath your arms and cradle your wrists (Fig. 61a).

Slowly straighten at the knees and waist, while your partner slowly pushes up, elevating your wrists (Fig. 61b). Hold at peak for 10 seconds, then release.

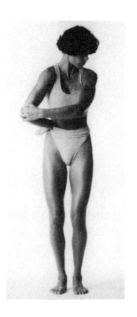

SIDE/REAR SHOULDER STRETCH
target: posterior & lateral deltoid heads

In a standing position, bend your right elbow and brace the back of your wrist in the hollow between your ribcage and the crest of your hip. Grasping it just above the elbow with your free hand, gently pull downward across your body (Fig. 62). When you reach maximum stretch, maintain pressure for about five seconds, then slowly release. Keep your shoulder down throughout. Repeat with other arm.

THE PROGRAM:
How and When

CHAPTER THIRTEEN

THE ROUTINES

There are two types of routines in *Transfigure II*: **Expanded** and **Condensed**. It's up to you to select the approach that best addresses your goals. Here are guidelines to help you choose.

Condensed

The **Condensed** approach provides a short, intense, full upper-body workout aimed at general toning and shaping. Because it is constructed of back-to-back exercise groupings (called *supersets*) for opposing muscle pairs, it is geared to promote symmetrical development of all areas of the upper body. As a result, it doesn't provide the opportunity to concentrate on a certain area more than the others. It is a simple, fast, intense, and well-balanced approach.

Expanded

The **Expanded** routines offer a modular approach: each body area (chest, back, delts, biceps, triceps) has its own self-contained routine. This gives you more control over your results by allowing you to focus special attention on the areas you particularly want to work. It also allows you to split the routine up into two separate workouts done on different days to keep your daily workout time short. (The Schedule Chapter, beginning page 89, explains how best to set up a split program using the **Expanded** routines.)

Both **Condensed** and **Expanded** routines consist of a series of levels. These progress from easy to difficult. In addition, some of the levels in the **Expanded** routines are lettered, some are numbered. The lettered levels (e.g. "Level **A**") use only the weight of your body and elastic bands to provide resistance. These routine levels can be done anywhere. The numbered levels (e.g. "Level **1**") use gym equipment—barbells, dumbbells, and machines—to provide higher resistance and produce faster results.

To tone and shape, choose the highest resistance routine for which you have the equipment. The higher the resistance, the faster the results.

(Some of the routines have an asterisk by a level—e.g. "Level 3*". The levels above an asterisked level are extremely high intensity, and you don't need to use them unless you are bodybuilding.)

To bodybuild, you have only one choice: use gym equipment. (Note to the nonbodybuilder: It's not the routine so much as the use of it that makes the difference between bodybuilding and toning. The bodybuilder must train at a much higher level of intensity, always striving to increase weight lifted, always working to keep pace at a maximum, as well as manipulating caloric intake, sleep, and other factors. Using gym equipment will not result in greater muscularity than you want; it will simply allow you to achieve your ideal shape more quickly.)

R e s t   B e t w e e n   S e t s

Allow no more than 10 to 15 seconds between sets of an exercise. Don't rest at *all* between the last set of one exercise and the first set of the next. During a single-arm exercise, alternate sets for left and right arms without resting.

S u p e r s e t s

Both **Condensed** and **Expanded** routines use **supersets**. A *superset* is two exercises performed back-to-back without rest.*

For example, *Level 1, Condensed* calls for two supersets of Supine Bench Presses and Close-Grip Pull-Downs. Each superset consists of a set of Supine Bench Presses followed immediately (without resting) by a set of Close-Grip Pull-Downs.

To perform two supersets, you would do: a set of Supine Bench Presses followed immediately by a set of Close-Grip Pull-Downs (that's the first superset); another set of Supine Bench Presses followed immediately by another set of Close-Grip Pull-Downs (that's the second superset).

If the note "@ arm" or "@ side" appears after the number of reps within the superset, like this...

- -

* Strictly speaking, a *superset* always involves two exercises for *opposing muscle groups* (biceps / triceps, quadriceps / hamstrings, etc.) performed back-to-back without rest. We use the term here in its more common form, referring to *any* two exercises performed back-to-back without rest.

3 Supersets . Triceps Dips . . . . 6-8 reps
Strap Triceps Extensions . . . 6-8 reps @ arm

...that means one of the exercises in the superset is a single-arm movement. You would do a set of the first exercise plus two sets of the second exercise—one for each arm—before starting the second superset (e.g., exercise A; exercise B, left arm, exercise B, right arm; exercise A; exercise B, left arm, exercise B, right arm; and so on).

Rest between sets: Allow no more than 20 to 40 seconds of rest between sets of an exercise. Don't rest *at all* between the last set of one exercise and the first set of the next. Don't rest between the exercises within a superset.

THE
CONDENSED
ROUTINES

Level 1

2 supersets . . Supine Bench Press . . . . 8-10 reps
Close-Grip Pull-Downs . . . . 8-10 reps

1 giant set . . Dumbbell Side Delt Raises . . . . 7 reps
Dumbbell Front Delt Raises . . . . . . 7 reps
Dumbbell Rear Delt Raises . . . . . . 7 reps

2 supersets . . Preacher Curls (w/dumbbells) . . 8-10 reps
Triceps Press-Downs . . . . 8-10 reps

2 sets . . . . . Hyperextensions . . . . .12-15 reps

Level 2 *

2 supersets . . Supine Bench Press . . . . 8-10 reps
Close-Grip Pull-Downs . . . . 8-10 reps

2 supersets . . Pec Flyes . . . . 8-10 reps
Standing One-Hand Rows . 8-10 reps @ arm

3 giant sets . . Dumbbell Side Delt Raises . . . . 7 reps
Dumbbell Front Delt Raises . . . . . . 7 reps
Dumbbell Rear Delt Raises . . . . . . 7 reps

2 supersets . . Preacher Curls (w/dumbbells) . . 8-10 reps
Triceps Press-Downs . . . . 8-10 reps

2 sets . . . . . Hyperextensions . . . . 12-15 reps

Level 3

2 supersets . . Supine Bench Press . . . . 6-8 reps
HFL Decline Rows . . . . 6-8 reps

2 supersets . . Pec Flyes . . . . 6-8 reps
Close-Grip Pull-Downs . . . . 6-8 reps

3 giant sets . . Dumbbell Side Delt Raises . . . . . . 7 reps
Dumbbell Front Delt Raises . . . . . 7 reps
Dumbbell Rear Delt Raises . . . . . 7 reps

2 supersets . . Preacher Curls (w/dumbbells) . . . 6-8 reps
Triceps Press-Downs . . . . 6-8 reps

2 supersets . . Seated Dumbbell Curls . . . . 6-8 reps
Triceps Kick-Backs . . . . 6-8 reps

2 sets . . . . . Hyperextensions . . . . 12-15 reps

Level 4

3 supersets . . Supine Bench Press . . . . 6-8 reps
HFL Decline Rows . . . . 6-8 reps

3 supersets . . Pec Flyes . . . . 6-8 reps
Close-Grip Pull-Downs . . . . 6-8 reps

3 giant sets . . Dumbbell Side Delt Raises . . . . . . 7 reps
Dumbbell Front Delt Raises . . . . . 7 reps
Dumbbell Rear Delt Raises . . . . . 7 reps

3 supersets . . Preacher Curls (w/cable) . . . . . . 6-8 reps
Lying French Press . . . . 6-8 reps

3 supersets . . Seated Dumbbell Curls . . . . 6-8 reps
Triceps Kick-Backs . . . . 6-8 reps

2 sets . . . . . Hyperextensions . . . . 12-15 reps

THE
EXPANDED
ROUTINES

Chest

Level A

3 sets . . . . . Kneeling Push-Ups . . . . 8-10 reps

Level B

2 sets . . . . . Kneeling Push-Ups . . . . 8-10 reps

2 sets . . . . . Decline Kneeling Push-Ups . . . . 8-10 reps

Level C

3 sets . . . . . Kneeling Push-Ups . . . . 8-10 reps

2 sets . . . . . One-Arm Side Push-Ups . . . . 8-10 reps

3 sets . . . . . Decline Kneeling Push-Ups . . . . 8-10 reps

Level 1

3 sets . . . . . Supine Bench Press . . . . 8-10 reps

Level 2

2 sets . . . . . Supine Bench Press . . . . 8-10 reps

2 set . . . . . Incline Bench Press . . . . 8-10 reps

Level 3

3 sets . . . . . Supine Bench Press . . . . 8-10 reps

3 sets . . . . . Incline Bench Press . . . . 8-10 reps

1 set . . . . . Pec Deck Flyes . . . . 8-10 reps

Level 4

3 sets . . . . . Supine Bench Press . . . . 6-8 reps

2 sets . . . . . Incline Bench Press . . . . 6-8 reps

1 set . . . . . Incline Pec Flyes . . . . 6-8 reps

1 set . . . . . Upper-Pec Cable Pulls . . . . 6-8 reps

T r i c e p s

Level A

3 sets . . . . . Kneeling Push-Ups, triceps position 10-12 reps

Level B

3 supersets . . Kneeling Push-Ups, triceps position 10-12 reps
. . . . Strap Triceps Extensions . . . . 6-8 reps

Level 1

3 sets . . . . . Triceps Press-Downs . . . . 8-10 reps

Level 2

2 supersets . . Triceps Press-Downs . . . . 8-10 reps
Kneeling Push-Ups, triceps position 8-10 reps

Level 3

3 supersets . . Triceps Press-Downs . . . . 8-10 reps
Kneeling Push-Ups, triceps position 8-10 reps

2 sets . . . . . Triceps Kick-Backs . . . . 6-8 reps

Level 4

3 supersets . . Triceps Press-Downs . . . . 8-10 reps
Kneeling Push-Ups, triceps position 8-10 reps

2 sets . . . . . Triceps Kick-Backs . . . . 6-8 reps

1 set . . . . . One-Hand Reverse-Grip Press Downs . . . .
. . . . 6-8 reps @ hand

Level 5

3 supersets . . Triceps Press-Downs . . . . 6-8 reps
Machine (or Chair) Dips . . . . 6-8 reps

2 sets . . . . . Triceps Kick-Backs . . . . 6-8 reps

1 set . . . . . One-Hand Reverse-Grip Press Downs . . . .
. . . . 6-8 reps @ hand

Back

Level A

3 sets . . . . . Supine Pull-Ups . . . . 8-10 reps

Level B

2 sets . . . . . Strap Seated Rows, low . . . . . . 8-10 reps

2 sets . . . . . Strap Seated Rows, high . . . . . . 8-10 reps

Level 1

3 sets . . . . . Close-Grip Pull-Downs . . . . 8-10 reps

2 sets . . . . . Hyperextensions . . . . 12-15 reps

Level 2 *

2 sets . . . . . Close-Grip Pull-Downs . . . . 8-10 reps

2 sets . . . . . Wide-Grip Pull-Downs . . . . 6-8 reps

2 sets . . . . . Hyperextensions . . . . 10-12 reps

Level 3

2 supersets . . Scapular Rolls . . . . 6-8 reps
Close-Grip Pull-Downs . . . . 8-10 reps

2 sets . . . . . Seated One-Hand Rows . . 8-10 reps @ side

1 set . . . . . Wide-Grip Pull-Downs . . . . 6-8 reps

2 sets . . . . . Hyperextensions . . . . 10-12 reps

Level 4

3 supersets . . Scapular Rolls . . . . 6-8 reps
Close-Grip Pull-Downs . . . . 6-8 reps

3 sets . . . . . HFL Decline Rows . . . . 6-8 reps

2 sets . . . . . Close-Grip Pull-Ups . . . . 6-8 reps

1 set . . . . . Seated One-Hand Rows . . . 6-8 reps @ side

2 sets . . . . . Hyperextensions . . . . 10-12 reps

Biceps

Level A

3 sets . . . . . Strap Curls . . . . 6-8 reps

Level 1

3 sets . . . . . Preacher Curls (w/dumbbells) . . . 6-8 reps

Level 2

3 sets . . . . . Preacher Curls (w/dumbbells) . . . 6-8 reps

2 sets . . . . . Standing Supinated
Dumbbell Curls . . . . 8-10 reps

Level 3 *

3 sets . . . . . Preacher Curls (w/cable) . . . . . . 6-8 reps

2 sets . . . . . Standing Supinated
Dumbbell Curls . . . . 8-10 reps

Level 4

3 sets . . . . . Preacher Curls (w/cable) . . . . . . 6-8 reps

2 sets . . . . . Seated Dumbbell Curls . . . . 6-8 reps

2 sets . . . . . Standing Supinated
Dumbbell Curls . . . . 8-10 reps

Deltoids

Level A

2 giant sets . . Strap Side Delt Raises . . . . 7 reps
Strap Front Delt Raises . . . . 7 reps
Bow-and-Arrows (Rear Delts) . . . . . 7 reps

Level 1

2 giant sets . . Dumbbell Side Delt Raises . . . . 7 reps
Dumbbell Front Delt Raises . . . . . . 7 reps
Dumbbell Rear Delt Raises . . . . . . 7 reps

Level 2*

3 giant sets . . Dumbbell Side Delt Raises . . . . 7 reps
Dumbbell Front Delt Raises . . . . . . 7 reps
Dumbbell Rear Delt Raises . . . . . . 7 reps

Level 3

2 giant sets . . Dumbbell Side Delt Raises . . . . 7 reps
Dumbbell Front Delt Raises . . . . . . 7 reps
Dumbbell Rear Delt Raises . . . . . . 7 reps
Behind-the-Neck Press . . . . 6-8 reps

Level 3 (with Machines)

2 giant sets . . Machine Side Delt Raises . . . . 7 reps
Machine Front Delt Raises . . . . 7 reps
Dumbbell Rear Delt Raises . . . . . . 7 reps
Behind-the-Neck Press . . . . 6-8 reps

CHAPTER FOURTEEN

THE
ROUTINES,
ILLUSTRATED

L
E
V
E
L

1

Supine Bench Press
8-10 reps

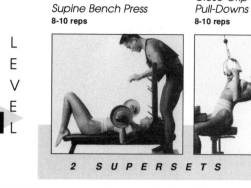

Close-Grip Pull-Downs
8-10 reps

2   S U P E R S E T S

Dumbbell Side Delt Raises
7 reps

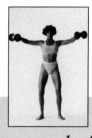

Dumbbell Front Delt Raises
7 reps

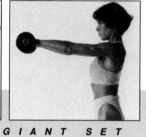

Dumbbell Rear Delt Raises
7 reps

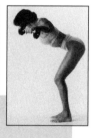

1   G I A N T   S E T

Preacher Curls (w/dumbbells)
8-10 reps

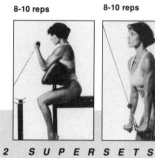

Triceps Press-Downs
8-10 reps

2   S U P E R S E T S

L
E
V
E
L

2

Supine Bench Press
6-8 reps

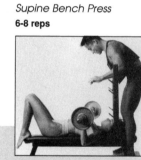

Close-Grip Pull-Downs
8-10 reps

2   S U P E R S E T S

Dumbbell Side Delt Raises
7 reps

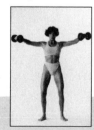

Dumbbell Front Delt Raises
7 reps

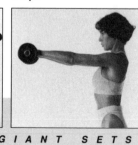

Dumbbell Rear Delt Raises
7 reps

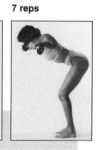

3   G I A N T   S E T S

THE ROUTINES
ILLUSTRATED
• c o n d e n s e d •

Hyperextensions
2 sets / 12-15 reps

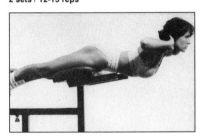

Pec Flyes
8-10 reps

*Standing
One-Hand Rows*
8-10 reps

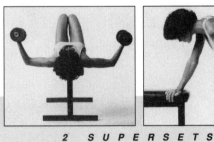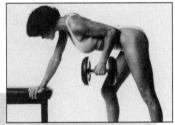

2 S U P E R S E T S

*Preacher Curls
(w/dumbbells)*
8-10 reps

*Triceps
Press-Downs*
8-10 reps

Hyperextensions
2 sets / 12-15 reps

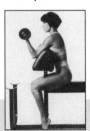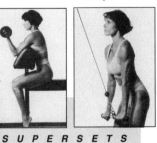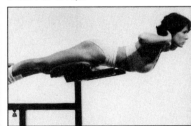

2 S U P E R S E T S

Supine Bench Press
6-8 reps

HFL Decline Rows
6-8 reps

L
E
V
E
L

3

2 S U P E R S E T S

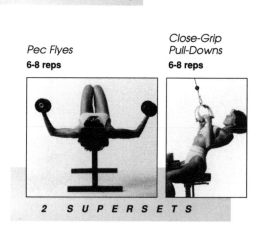

Pec Flyes
6-8 reps

Close-Grip Pull-Downs
6-8 reps

2 S U P E R S E T S

THE ROUTINES
I L L U S T R A T E D
• c o n d e n s e d •

*Dumbbell
Side Delt Raises*
7 reps

*Dumbbell
Front Delt Raises*
7 reps

*Dumbbell
Rear Delt Raises*
7 reps

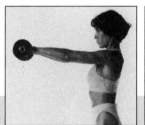
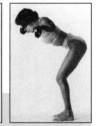

3   G I A N T   S E T S

*Preacher Curls
(w/dumbbells)*
6-8 reps

*Triceps
Press-Downs*
6-8 reps

*Seated
Dumbbell Curls*
6-8 reps

Triceps Kick-Backs
6-8 reps

Hyperextensions
2 sets / 12-15 reps

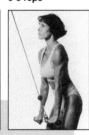
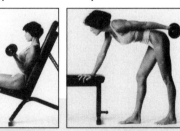
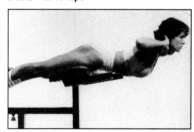

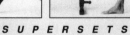

2   S U P E R S E T S   **2   S U P E R S E T S**

4

Supine Bench Press
6-8 reps

HFL Decline Rows
6-8 reps

Pec Flyes
6-8 reps

Close-Grip
Pull-Downs
6-8 reps

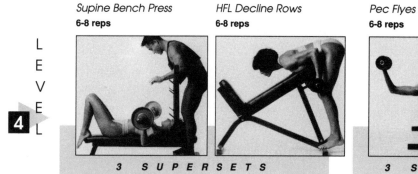

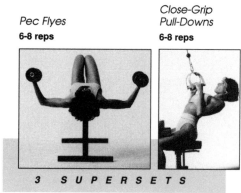

3   S U P E R S E T S

3   S U P E R S E T S

Dumbbell
Side Delt Raises
7 reps

Dumbbell
Front Delt Raises
7 reps

Dumbbell
Rear Delt Raises
7 reps

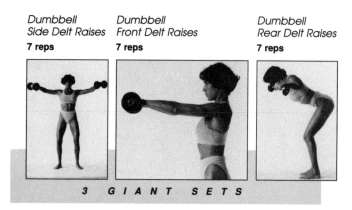

3   G I A N T   S E T S

THE ROUTINES
ILLUSTRATED
• c o n d e n s e d •

Preacher Bench
Curls (with
cable)
6-8 reps

Lying French Press
6-8 reps

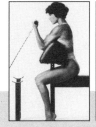
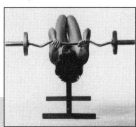

3   S U P E R S E T S

Seated
Dumbbell Curls
6-8 reps

Triceps Kick-Backs
6-8 reps

Hyperextensions
2 sets / 12-15 reps

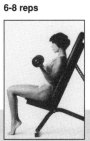
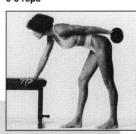
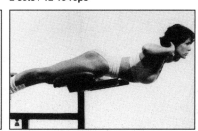

3   S U P E R S E T S

Kneeling Push-Ups
3 sets / 8-10 reps

L
E
V
E
L

A ▶

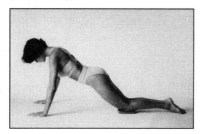

Kneeling Push-Ups
2 sets / 8-10 reps

L
E
V
E
L

B ▶

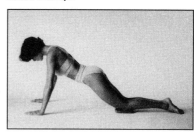

Kneeling Push-Ups
3 sets / 8-10 reps

One-Arm Side Push-Ups
2 sets / 8-10 reps

L
E
V
E
L

C ▶

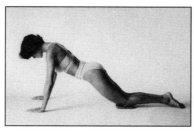
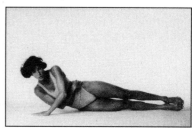

Supine Bench Press
3 sets / 8-10 reps

L
E
V
E
L

1 ▶

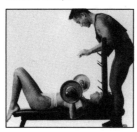

Supine Bench Press
2 sets / 8-10 reps

*Incline
Bench Press*
2 sets / 8-10 reps

L
E
V
E
L

2 ▶

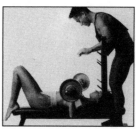
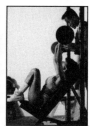

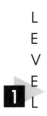

Decline Kneeling Push-Ups
(or) Tent Push-Ups
2 sets / 8-10 reps

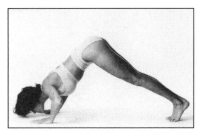

Decline Kneeling Push-Ups
(or) Tent Push-Ups
3 sets / 8-10 reps

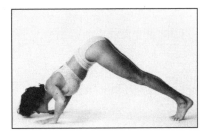

THE ROUTINES
ILLUSTRATED
• c h e s t •

L E V E L **3**

Supine Bench Press
3 sets / 8-10 reps

Incline Bench Press
3 sets / 8-10 reps

Pec Deck Flyes
1 set / 8-10 reps

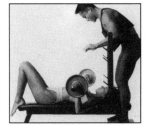
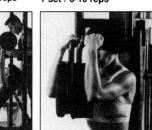

L E V E L **4**

Supine Bench Press
3 sets / 6-8 reps

Incline Bench Press
2 sets / 6-8 reps

Incline Pec Flyes
1 set / 6-8 reps

Upper-Pec Cable Pulls
1 set / 6-8 reps

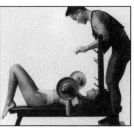
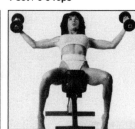
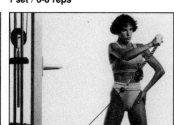

Kneeling Push-Ups, Triceps Position
3 sets / 10-12 reps

L
E
V
E
A L

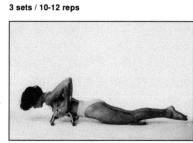

Kneeling Push-Ups, Triceps Position
10-12 reps

Strap Triceps Extensions
6-8 reps

L
E
V
B E
L

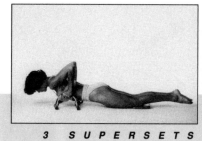 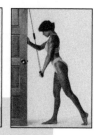

3 S U P E R S E T S

Triceps Press-Downs
3 Sets / 8-10 reps

L
E
V
E
1 L

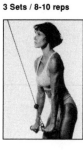

Triceps Press-Downs
8-10 reps

Kneeling Push-ups, Triceps Position
8-10 reps

L
E
V
2 E
L

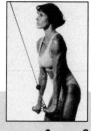 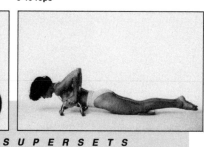

2 S U P E R S E T S

Triceps Press-Downs
8-10 reps

Kneeling Push-ups, Triceps Position
8-10 reps

Triceps Kick-Backs
2 sets / 6-8 reps

1-Hand Reverse-Grip Press-Downs
1 set / 6-8 reps @

L
E
V
E
4 L

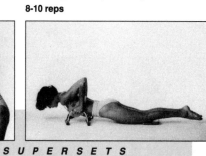 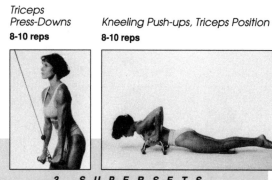 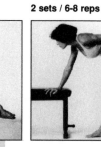 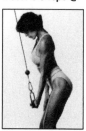

3 S U P E R S E T S

THE ROUTINES
ILLUSTRATED
• triceps •

LEVEL **3**

Triceps Press-Downs
8-10 reps

Kneeling Push-ups, Triceps Position
8-10 reps

Triceps Kick-Backs
2 sets / 6-8 reps

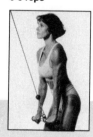 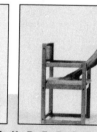 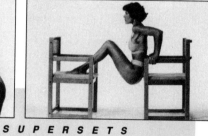

3 SUPERSETS

LEVEL 5

Triceps Press-Downs
6-8 reps

Machine (or Chair) Dips
6-8 reps

Triceps Kick-Backs
2 sets / 6-8 reps

1-Hand Reverse-Grip Press-Downs
1 set / 6-8 reps ea.

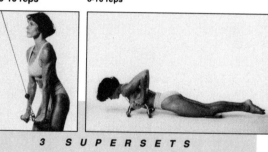 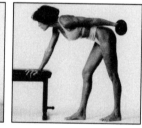 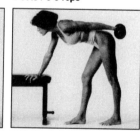 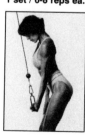

3 SUPERSETS

Supine Pull-Ups
3 sets / 8-10 reps

L
E
V
E
L

A

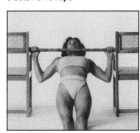

Strap Seated Rows, Low
2 sets / 8-10 reps

Strap Seated Rows, High
2 sets / 8-10 reps

L
E
V
E
L

B

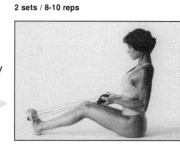

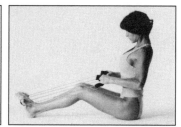

*Close-Grip
Pull-Downs*
3 Sets / 8-10 reps

Hyperextensions
2 Sets / 12-15 reps

L
E
V
E
L

1

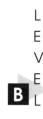

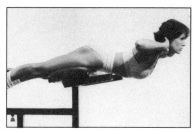

*Close-Grip
Pull-Downs*
2 sets / 8-10 reps

L
E
V
E
L

2

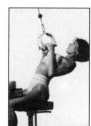

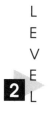

If you are doing Level 1 or Level 2 and you would like
to increase the intensity without moving up to the next
level, superset Close-Grip Pull-Downs with Scapular
Rolls (see Level 3 for example).

Scapular Rolls
6-8 reps

*Close-Grip
Pull-Downs*
8-10 reps

L
E
V
E
L

3

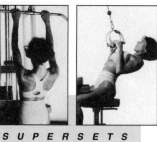

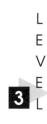

2   S U P E R S E T S

Scapular Rolls
6-8 reps

*Close-Grip
Pull-Downs*
6-8 reps

HFL Decline Rows
3 sets / 6-8 reps

L
E
V
E
L

4

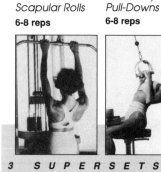

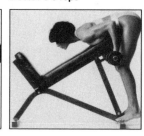

3   S U P E R S E T S

THE ROUTINES
ILLUSTRATED
• back •

Wide-Grip Pull-Downs
2 sets / 6-8 reps

Hyperextensions
2 Sets / 10-12 reps

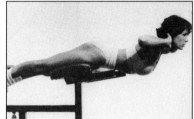

Seated One-Hand Rows
2 sets / 8-10 reps per side

Wide-Grip Pull-Downs
1 sets / 6-8 reps

Hyperextensions
2 sets / 10-12 reps

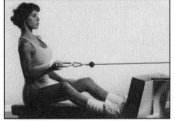

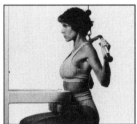

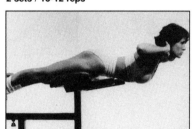

*Close-Grip
Pull-Ups*
2 sets / 6-8 reps

Seated One-Hand Rows
1 set / 6-8 reps per side

Hyperextensions
2 sets / 10-12 reps

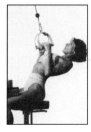

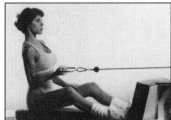

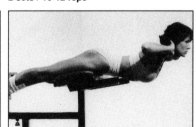

Strap Curls

3 Sets / 6-8 reps

L
E
V
E
L

A ▶

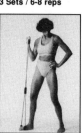

*Preacher Curls
(with
Dumbbells)*

3 Sets / 6-8 reps

L
E
V
E
L

1 ▶

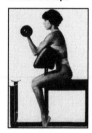

*Preacher Curls
(with
Dumbbells)*

3 Sets / 6-8 reps

*Standing
Supinated
Dumbbell Curls*

2 Sets / 8-10 reps

L
E
V
E
L

2 ▶

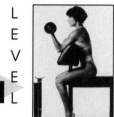
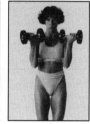

*Preacher Curls
(with Cable)*

3 Sets / 6-8 reps

*Standing
Supinated
Dumbbell Curls*

2 Sets / 8-10 reps

L
E
V
E
L

3 ▶

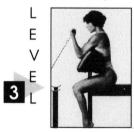
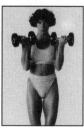

THE ROUTINES
ILLUSTRATED
• b i c e p s

Preacher Curls   *Seated*   *Standing*
(with cable)   *Dumbbell Curls*   *Supinated*
                                           Dumbbell Curls

3 sets / 6-8 reps   **2 sets / 6-8 reps**   **2 sets / 8-10 reps**

L
E
V
E
L

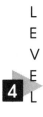
4

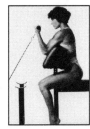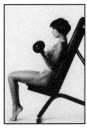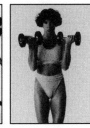

*Strap
Side Delt Raises*
7 reps

*Strap
Front Delt Raises*
7 reps

*Bow-and-Arrows
(Rear Delts)*
7 reps

L
E
V
E
L

A

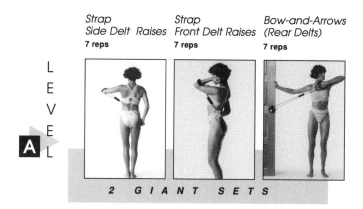

2 G I A N T S E T S

*Dumbbell
Side Delt Raises*
7 reps

*Dumbbell
Front Delt Raises*
7 reps

*Dumbbell
Rear Delt Raises*
7 reps

L
E
V
E
L

1

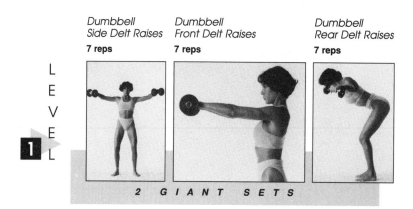

2 G I A N T S E T S

*Dumbbell
Side Delt Raises*
7 reps

*Dumbbell
Front Delt Raises*
7 reps

*Dumbbell
Rear Delt Raises*
7 reps

*Behind-the-
Neck Press*
6-8 reps

L
E
V
E
L

3

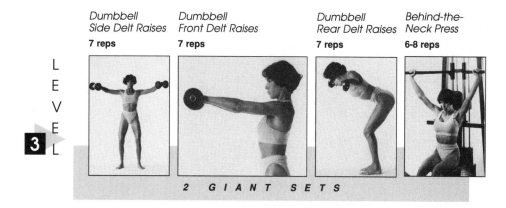

2 G I A N T S E T S

THE ROUTINES
ILLUSTRATED
• deltoids •

LEVEL 2

Dumbbell Side Delt Raises — **7 reps**
Dumbbell Front Delt Raises — **7 reps**
Dumbbell Rear Delt Raises — **7 reps**

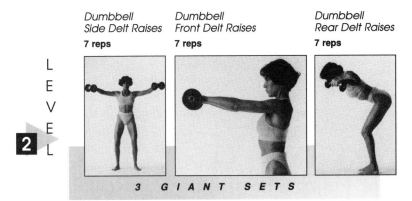

3 GIANT SETS

LEVEL 3 (WITH MACHINES)

Machine Side Delt Raises — **6-8 reps**
Machine Front Delt Raises — **7 reps**
Dumbbell Rear Delt Raises — **7 reps**
Behind-the-Neck Press — **6-8 reps**

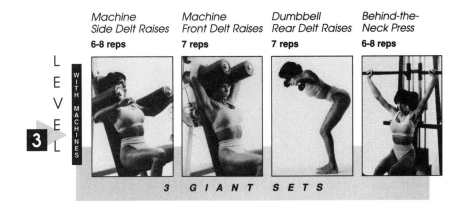

3 GIANT SETS

CHAPTER FIFTEEN

THE SCHEDULE

Condensed

Using the **Transfigure II, Condensed** routines is an intense, quick way to tone and shape your upper body. The routines are ideal if you have limited time to train. The're also ideal if you want to use resistance training to condition for other sports, such as racquetball. For fastest results, do the appropriate level three times per week, immediately after lower-body work.

Allow at least one rest day between workouts. You might, for example, work out Monday, Wednesday, and Friday. The specific days are not important; allowing a rest day between sessions is.

Don't do the routine more often than three times per week. If you do, you risk overtraining.* This can actually decrease your results.

Also, don't be in a hurry to move up through the levels. The idea is to get as much out of as little work as possible. As long as you are getting results with a particular level, stay with it. Move up only when you stop seeing improvement.

(It's impossible to tell you exactly when to move from one level to the next. That is largely a matter of "feel." Most people find they can progress through the lower levels fairly quickly—spending just a few weeks on each. Generally they reach an upper level that becomes their "regular" workout, and stay with that level for a long time before making the next move up.)

Expanded

Transfigure II, Expanded is a powerful system of high-resistance, low-repetition training. It takes a bit longer than the **Condensed** approach, but ultimately will produce greater improvement. Because the **Expanded** approach is more flexible than the

. . . .

* **Overtraining** is a state in which the body can no longer adapt to the stress imposed on it by exercise.

Condensed one, it requires a little more thought in putting together your weekly schedule.

At lower levels of the routines (which involve fewer sets and therefore don't take as long to perform), you may find it convenient to work all parts of the upper body on the same day, as in the **Condensed** routines. The five modules (chest, back, delts, biceps, triceps) should always be arranged in two pairs of opposing groups: chest/back, and biceps/triceps. The area on which you want to concentrate should be placed first in each pair. The delt routine falls between the two pairs.

The four possible combinations are:

1—Back/Chest, Delts, Biceps/Triceps
2—Back/Chest, Delts, Triceps/Biceps
3—Chest/Back, Delts, Biceps/Triceps
4—Chest/Back, Delts, Triceps/Biceps

For example, if your main areas of concern were chest and triceps, then option #4 would be your best choice.

Interdependency rule. Notice that _either_ chest or back always comes first in the routine. The reason for this is that muscle groups cooperate to perform certain exercises. It's almost impossible, for instance, to work back or chest without involving the muscles of the arms. If you were to start off with arm exercises, you'd run the risk of tiring those muscles to the point where they would limit the chest and back work you could do afterward. To avoid this problem, the basic rule is: _work from the center of the body outward_.

Modifying the routines. Exercise order within routines is critical. If you decide to substitute exercises within the routines in this course, there is another rule, related to the concept of interdependency, to keep in mind: When sequencing several exercises for the _same_ bodypart, _do multi-joint exercises first_. Multi-joint exercises are the ones most likely to promote _functional strength_, because they involve a coordinated effort of several muscles, and because they are more effective when performed with more weight.

For example, when working the chest, you would do Bench Press, a multi-joint chest exercise, before Peck Deck, a single-joint chest exercise.

Intermediate and Advanced Splits. As you move through the levels of your routine, you may at some point decide to split up the work over several days, to keep your daily workout time to a minimum. Here are two possibilities:

Four-Day Split

*Day 1—**Transfigure I** (Lower Body)*
*Day 2—**Transfigure II** (Upper Body)*
Day 3—rest
*Day 4—**Transfigure I** (Lower Body)*
*Day 5—**Transfigure II** (Upper Body)*
Day 6—rest
Day 7—rest

Five-Day, Three-Week Split

*Week 1.   Day 1—**Transfigure I** (Lower Body)*
Day 2—Back, biceps, rear delts
Day 3—Chest, triceps, side and front delts
Day 4—rest
*Day 5—**Transfigure I** (Lower Body)*
Day 6—Back, biceps, rear delts
Day 7—rest

Week 2.   Day 1—Chest, triceps, side and front delts
*Day 2—**Transfigure I** (Lower Body)*
Day 3—Back, biceps, rear delts
Day 4—rest
Day 5—Chest, triceps, side and front delts
*Day 6—**Transfigure I** (Lower Body)*
Day 7—rest

Week 3.   Day 1—Back, biceps, rear delts
Day 2—Chest, triceps, side and front delts
*Day 3—**Transfigure I** (Lower Body)*
Day 4—rest
Day 5—Back, biceps, rear delts
Day 6—Chest, triceps, side and front delts
Day 7—rest

...then start the cycle over.

Notice that in the five-day schedule, deltoid exercises are divided between chest and back days. This is because the front and side portions of the deltoids are more closely aligned in action with the pectorals and triceps; the rear deltoid more so with the back muscles.

Again, don't be in a hurry to move up through the levels. As long as you are getting results with a particular level, stay with it.

Good luck—and happy training!

GLOSSARY

glossary

Abduction, shoulder:
raising your arm out to the side.

Adduction, shoulder:
bringing your arm down to your side from an abducted position.

Balanced Development:
proportional development of strength in each of the muscles of an opposing muscle group pair at a joint (e.g. biceps/triceps).

Delts:
the deltoid muscle of the shoulder, consisting of three "heads" or sections: the <u>anterior</u> deltoid, which raises the arm forward; the <u>lateral</u> deltoid, which raises the arm to the side; and the <u>posterior</u> deltoid, which raises the arm to the rear.

Extension, elbow:
straightening the elbow.

Extension, shoulder:
starting with your arm pointing straight forward, bringing your arm down to your side.

Fan-shaped muscle:
A muscle whose fibers converge at one end and diverge at the other and therefore don't all pull in the same direction. Examples: the pecs, traps, and lats. The line of force for a fan-shaped muscle can change depending on which muscle fibers in the fan are activated.

Flexion, elbow:
bending the elbow.

Flexion, shoulder:
bringing the arm up and forward.

Functional Strength:
the ability of the body to bring a coordinated muscular effort to bear on external resistance in everyday situations.

Hyperextension:
moving beyond fully straightened. Example: hyperextending the back means bending backward beyond the point where the torso is fully upright.

Lats:
the latissimus dorsi, a fan-shaped muscle of the back. Pulls the arm down and back.

Leverage:
mechanical advantage provided by position.

Optimization:
maximizing output for a given input

Overloading:
forcing a muscle to act against resistance greater than that which it can easily overcome, to encourage growth.

Pecs:
the pectoralis major and minor, fan-shaped muscles of the chest. The pectoralis major can be thought of as consisting of three muscle segments—the upper pecs, which pulls the arm up across the chest; the middle pecs, which pulls the arm straight across the chest; and the lower pecs, which pulls the arm down across the chest. The pectoralis minor pulls the shoulder blade down and forward.

Prime Mover:
the main muscle or muscle group responsible for a given movement.

Pronation, forearm:
rotation of the forearm resulting in the hand facing palm down.

Straight muscle:
a muscle whose fibers all run in the same direction, and which therefore has only one line of force.

Resistance:
the opposition to motion resulting from the combined effect of load and leverage.

Superset:
two exercises performed back-to-back without rest.

Supine:
lying on your back.

Supination, forearm:
rotation of the forearm resulting in the hand facing palm up.

Teres group:
the teres major and teres minor, two muscles of the back which pull the arm toward the shoulder blade.

Target:
the muscle or muscles that a given exercise primarily aims to work.

Tension:
muscular contractile force.

Timing (or pace):
the combination of rep speed, rests between sets, and rests between exercises.

Traps:
the trapezius, a fan-shaped muscle of the back.